THE EYE
AND ITS DISORDERS
IN THE ELDERLY

The Eye
and its Disorders
in the Elderly

Edited by

F. I. Caird DM FRCP

David Cargill Professor of Geriatric Medicine, University of Glasgow

and

John Williamson MD, FRCS

Consultant Ophthalmologist, Southern General Hospital, Glasgow

Bristol
1986

○ **John Wright & Sons Ltd.** 1986

Published by

John Wright & Sons Ltd. Techno House, Redcliffe Way, Bristol BS1 6NX

British Library Cataloguing in Publication Data

Caird, F. I.
  The eye and its disorders in the elderly.
  1. Geriatric ophthalmology
  I. Title   II. Williamson, John, *1935–*
  618.97'77   RE48.2.A5

ISBN 0 7236 0706 0

Typeset by
Severntype Repro Services Ltd,
Market Street, Wotton-under-Edge, Glos

Printed in Great Britain by
John Wright & Sons (Printing) Ltd
at The Stonebridge Press,
Bristol BS4 5NU

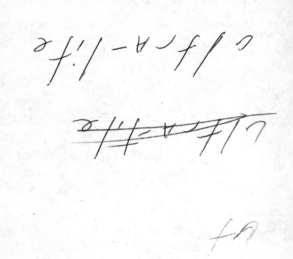

Preface

The combination of an ageing population and the fact that many serious eye diseases increase dramatically in frequency with age makes it essential that those who are interested in the medicine of old age in its broadest sense should be aware of the importance of diseases of the eye. It is in the best interests of elderly patients that geriatricians should know more about ophthalmology, and that ophthalmologists should know more about ageing and the medicine of old age. Multiple pathology in a single patient is now recognized as a commonplace, but nowhere is the further development of this concept to cover multiple pathology in a single organ better illustrated than in the eye. The purpose of the present volume is to bring together the views of experts so as both to give an account of the present state of scientific knowledge, and also most importantly to provide practical advice on the numerous problems of management encountered in everyday practice.

It is a pleasure to thank Mrs M. Smith for secretarial skills, Mrs M. Williamson for the practical support to both of us which made the editing of this volume so enjoyable, and Mr Roy Baker of John Wright & Sons Ltd for his assistance and guidance with the practical problems of a multi-author volume, and for his tolerance of editorial delays.

F. I. C.
J. W.

Contributors

B. Ashworth MD FRCP
Consultant Neurologist
Northern General Hospital, Edinburgh

T. Barrie MB FRCS
Consultant Ophthalmologist
Gartnavel General Hospital, Glasgow

F. I. Caird DM FRCP
David Cargill Professor of Geriatric Medicine
University of Glasgow

Hector B. Chawla FRCS
Consultant Ophthalmologist
Royal Infirmary, Edinburgh

A. L. Crombie MB FRCS
Professor of Ophthalmology
University of Newcastle upon Tyne

S. I. Davidson FRCS
Director of Studies, Department of Ophthalmology
University of Liverpool

J. Dudgeon MB FRCS DO
Consultant Ophthalmologist
Tennent Institute of Ophthalmology, University of Glasgow

R. C. Eagle jun. MD
Assistant Professor of Ophthalmology
University of Pennsylvania School of Medicine

H. B. Kennedy MB FRCS
Consultant Ophthalmologist
Southern General Hospital, Glasgow

M. F. Marmor MD
Associate Professor of Ophthalmology/Surgery
Stanford University Medical Center, California

S. P. Meadows MD BSc FRCP
Consulting Physician, Moorfields Eye Hospital
National Hospital, Queen Square and Westminster Hospital

C. I. Phillips MD PhD DPH MSc FRCS DO FBOA (Hon)
Professor of Ophthalmology
University of Edinburgh

I. G. Rennie MB FRCS
Lecturer, Department of Ophthalmology
University of Liverpool

J. S. Shilling FRCS
Consultant Ophthalmologist
St Thomas' Hospital, London

John Williamson MD FRCS
Consultant Ophthalmologist
Southern General Hospital, Glasgow

W. Wilson MB FRCS DO
Consultant Ophthalmologist
Royal Infirmary, Glasgow

M. Yanoff MD FACS
Chairman, Department of Ophthalmology
University of Pennsylvania School of Medicine

Contents

1. EPIDEMIOLOGY OF OCULAR DISORDERS IN OLD AGE
John Williamson and F. I. Caird

The uses of epidemiology include the measurement of the size of a clinical problem, as a guide to planning and assistance in the monitoring of success and failure of medical and other measures, and the provision of theories of aetiology for different conditions. Difficulties include the problems of defining and recording a population base, the practical problems of definition and recording of data (WHO (1966) recognizes no fewer than 65 definitions of blindness), and diagnostic and other medical fashions. The statistics of blindness, which may be likened to ocular death certificates, are no exception.

BLINDNESS STATISTICS

There are slight variations between countries in their definition of blindness, and a much greater variation in the reasons for and the advantages of registration, which bear on the likelihood of the completeness of any statistics. In most countries blindness registration is not compulsory, and carries with it few advantages. In others, such as the United Kingdom, registration is known to be incomplete, with up to a third of elderly women who qualify for registration unregistered (Graham et al., 1968). Registration may be refused, often because of the necessity of prior disclosure of personal finances, or patients may be placed on the Blind Register while awaiting treatment in order to gain the benefits of the Register, and then removed after successful treatment. This will clearly affect the apparent prevalence of blindness due for instance to cataract. Changing diagnostic fashions, particularly perhaps in the field of senile macular degeneration, are probably also important. Complexity, especially perhaps in the elderly, results from the existence of multiple causes of blindness, either different in the two eyes or combined in both; this is quite a common problem, and one so complicated as to defy rational description. Despite all these problems much useful information can be derived from blindness statistics on the incidence and prevalence of severe ocular disease leading to blindness.

The certification and registration of lesser degrees of visual impair-

1

ment is much less perfect. The definitions used are much more variable; registration is often linked to employment, and therefore does not apply to the elderly. Information of this kind, by comparison with that derived from blindness statistics, is virtually useless in the elderly. The determination of the effect of ocular diseases in causing lesser degrees of visual impairment than blindness must, in the elderly, rest almost entirely upon population studies (*see below*).

The most satisfactory and complete blindness statistics are probably those of England and Wales (Sorsby, 1972). They show a striking relation to age of the incidence of new registration as blind, with rates increasing from about 1/1000 per year at the age of 70 to 7/1000 per year at the age of 90 (*Fig.* 1.1). The age and sex specific incidence rates were stable throughout the 1960s; there is no evidence that there have been any significant changes since then, though in Scotland in 1980 there were more males than females registered over the age of 85 (Ghafour et al., 1983).

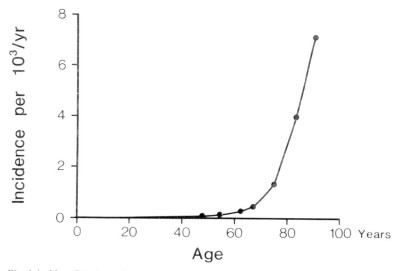

Fig. 1.1. New Blindness Registrations in England and Wales, 1968 (males: figures for females virtually identical; from Sorsby, 1972).

Since the incidence of blindness increases so dramatically with age, it is no surprise that the prevalence of a condition which does not carry an excess mortality (except for diabetic retinopathy) also increases with age: 48 per cent of men registered as blind, and 61 per cent of women, are over 70 years of age. The prevalence rate is about 2·5 per cent at age 85,

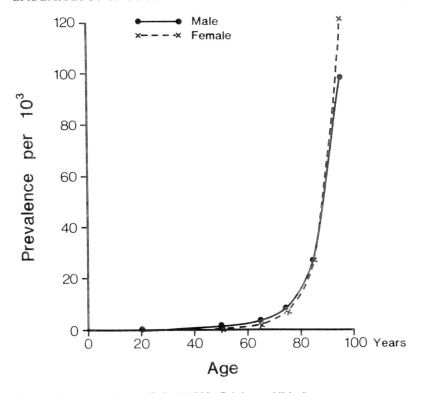

Fig. 1.2. Registered Blind in Oxford, 1966 (Caird, unpublished).

and as high as 10 per cent over the age of 90 (*Fig.* 1.2). It is therefore a common state of affairs, and one bearing very greatly on the rehabilitation of the elderly after any physical or mental illness (*see* Caird et al., 1983), and on their everyday life at home.

Conditions which cause blindness are of great importance to geriatricians. *Table* 1.1 shows the proportions of the various causes. The commonest is senile macular degeneration, but the several types of condition included under this heading are not adequately distinguished. However, all refer to conditions with a very close relation to old age, especially extreme old age, and only recently considered as treatable. Glaucoma and cataract are not peculiar to, though common, as causes of blindness in the elderly; they are together its second most common cause, and should be diligently sought by geriatricians since they are curable or preventable causes of loss of sight. Myopic chorioretinal degeneration remains a not uncommon cause of blindness, but is neither

Table 1.1. Causes of blindness in 506 eyes in persons registered blind over age 65 in Scotland (Ghafour et al., 1983)

Age	65–74	75–84	85+	65+
No. of eyes	214	216	76	506
Percent with:				
Senile macular lesions	26	48	49	39
Glaucoma	21	16	8	17
Cataract	11	9	30	13
Myopic chorioretinal degeneration	9	5	5	5
Diabetic retinopathy	5	7	—	7
Other	29	16	8	21

treatable nor preventable in our present state of knowledge. Diabetic retinopathy is relatively much more important in younger people, although over half of the patients blind from diabetic retinopathy are elderly (Caird et al., 1969); they make up a small percentage of the total elderly blind, owing to the predominance of other diseases.

Registration for blindness due to cataract is critically dependent on the effectiveness of local ophthalmological services and on the reasons for certification as stated above. The most reliable is likely to be from areas with good ophthalmic services where no one is placed on the blind register while awaiting operation, and the only patients certified as blind from cataract are those with complications of operation or those thought to be unfit for operation on medical or psychiatric grounds.

POPULATION STUDIES

Population surveys may be used to define the prevalence of both symptomatic and asymptomatic ocular disease, but careful scrutiny must be given to how the population study was defined, how it was recruited, what methods of examination were used, and also what definitions of given diseases were employed. Much the most satisfactory and comprehensive population study so far conducted in respect of ocular disease in the elderly is that in Framingham, Mass. (Kini et al., 1978; Sperduto and Seigel, 1980).

The wide variation in the lesions considered as resulting from senile macular degeneration makes it difficult to define and thus to establish its prevalence. However, in Framingham, it was reported as 35, 47, and 50 per cent at ages 51–64, 65–74, and 75–85 respectively (*Table* 1.2) visual symptoms were very much less common. It is thus clear that minor degrees of macular change are very common (but not universal), and that severer degrees producing symptoms are considerably less so. Never-

Table 1.2. Senile macular degeneration in the Framingham survey
(Kini et al., 1978; Sperduto and Seigel, 1980)

Age		52–64		65–74		75–85	
Sex		M	F	M	F	M	F
Prevalence	Total	39	32	46	48	49	50
Per cent	Early	19	16	18	24	13	14
	Moderate/severe	20	16	28	24	36	36
	Reduced visual acuity (6/9 or less)	2	1	9	13	24	30

Early: pigment disturbance or less than 10 drusen.
Moderate/severe: 10 or more drusen, elevated pigment layer or retina, or perimacular circinate exudates.

theless, these lesions represent the commonest single cause of blindness in old age (*Table* 1.1).

The statistics for the population prevalence of glaucoma are very sensitive to definition. Hollows and Graham (1966) found that intraocular pressure in the population, whether defined by applanation pressures or Schiotz readings, is affected by age, both pressures considerably rising with age (*Table* 1.3), and are higher at all ages in

Table 1.3. Prevalence per cent of ocular hypertension (intra-ocular pressure 21 mmHg or more on one occasion)
(*After* Hollows and Graham, 1966)

Age	M	F
40–9	6·3	6·6
50–9	6·7	11·7
60–4	8·8	15·6
65–9	10·4	12·0
70–4	11·8	18·6

women than men. The problem is very similar to that of the distribution of blood pressure, the majority of the population being 'normal', and a minority having pressures raised above an age-related upper limit of normal. The prevalence of ocular hypertension, defined as a pressure of 21 mmHg or more, rose with age from approximately 5 per cent at age 45 to 15 per cent in women and 10 per cent in men at age 70. Approximately a third of those with pressure of 21 mmHg or over but under 25 mmHg had ocular hypertension in one in three readings only, and so were not considered as confirmed. Confirmed ocular hypertension still showed an increase in frequency with age. The prevalence of true chronic simple glaucoma was however very much lower; thus, at the age of 75, confirmed ocular hypertension as defined was calculated as

Table 1.4. Senile lens changes in the Framingham study
(Kini et al., 1978; Sperduto and Seigel, 1980)

| Age | | 52–64 | | 65–74 | | 75–85 | |
Sex		M	F	M	F	M	F
Prevalence	Total	38	45	68	77	88	93
Per cent	Early	20	21	20	19	12	10
	Late	18	24	48	57	76	83
	Cataract	4	5	16	19	42	49

Early: lens vacuoles, water-clefts, spokes, or lamellar separations, on slit-lamp examination.
Late: cortical cuneiform opacities, decreased lucency of lens nucleus, posterior subcapsular or miscellaneous opacities.
Cataract: posterior or cortical lens changes or nuclear sclerosis, and visual acuity 6/9 or less, or aphakia.

being 19 times more common. It must be stressed that the term 'ocular hypertension' is a contentious one, and not accepted by all ophthalmologists. Differing definitions certainly make it difficult to compare these figures with those of the Framingham study (Kini et al., 1978); the latter shows a higher prevalence of raised intra-ocular pressure in males at all ages. Ocular hypertension leads to chronic simple glaucoma relatively rarely, and treatment must take this consideration into account. (See p. 85 for the epidemiology of glaucoma.)

The Framingham study shows conclusively the increase with age in senile cataract (defined as aphakia, or posterior or subcapsular lens changes or nuclear sclerosis, associated with a best corrected visual acuity of 6/9 or less); the prevalence is given as 5 per cent at age 52–64, 19 per cent at 65–74, and 46 per cent at age 75–85 (Table 1.4). The prevalence in the Edinburgh survey (Milne and Williamson, 1972)—22 per cent at ages from 62 to 79—is essentially similar.

There would appear to be few if any studies on the natural history of myopic chorioretinal atrophy, the fourth commonest cause of blindness in the elderly. It is generally believed that only those with myopia of high degree will develop this complication. Its importance as a cause of blindness is a clear demonstration of the effect of 'congenital' lesions in old age.

The prevalence of diabetic retinopathy is given in the Framingham study as 2, 3, and 7 per cent at ages 52–64, 65–74, 75–85, respectively. Again, definitions are difficult, especially in respect of the significance as diabetic of hard exudates alone, without the characteristic retinal haemorrhages or microaneurysms. These figures are, however, considerably above those given by Caird et al. (1969), but comparable to those in younger age groups. Nevertheless, there is no doubt of substantial variation from country to country in both the prevalence of diabetes itself, and of the frequency among diabetics of its various complications (see Caird et al., 1969).

OTHER METHODS

Operation statistics have been used to demonstrate the relation of cataract and age (Caird et al., 1965; Caird, 1973), but here many factors are involved before there can be any definite conclusions. The figures are affected by the efficiency and completeness of ophthalmological services in the area in question, the coverage of the target population, and what may be called the 'operation ratio', that is the proportion of patients fulfilling the ocular criteria for operation who are in fact operated upon. In cataract, although the operation ratio may well fall with age, the criteria for operation are in general the same in elderly men and women, though they differ from those applied to younger patients (Caird et al., 1965).

Admission statistics (e.g. Goldacre and Ingram, 1983) can by their nature only cover patients admitted to hospital, and are therefore only of value when admission to hospital is necessary, for instance for operation. Insofar as much ophthalmological practice, even in the elderly, is on an outpatient basis, they are likely to be of little value in many conditions.

SUMMARY

All these studies, though widely variable in their methods and in the weight that can be given to their results, show that ocular disease increases more or less exponentially with age, and thus that the very old are at a very considerable risk of one or more. They are thus of great importance to geriatricians, who must be alert to the problems presented, and aware of the early manifestations of those conditions that are amenable to treatment.

REFERENCES

Caird F. I. (1973) In: Pirie, A. (ed.), *The Human Lens in Relation to Cataract.* Amsterdam, ASP. p. 281.
Caird F. I., Hutchinson M. and Pirie A. (1965) *Br. J. Prev. Soc. Med.* **19**, 80.
Caird F. I., Kennedy R. D. and Williams B. O. (1983) *Practical Rehabilitation of the Elderly.* London, Pitman Medical.
Caird F. I., Pirie A. and Ramsell T. G. (1969) *Diabetes and the Eye.* Oxford, Blackwell Scientific Publications.
Ghafour I. M., Allan D. and Foulds W. S. (1983) *Br. J. Ophthalmol.* **67**, 209.
Goldacre M. J. and Ingram R. M. (1983) *Br. Med. J.* **286**, 1560.
Graham P. A., Wallace J., Welsby E. and Grace H. J. (1968) *Br. J. Prev. Soc. Med* **22**, 238.
Hollows F. C. and Graham P. A. (1966) *Br. J. Ophthalmol.* **50**, 570.
Kini M. M., Leibowitz H. M., Colton T. et al. (1978) *Am. J. Ophthalmol.* **85**, 28.
Milne J. A. and Williamson J. (1972) *Geront. Clin.* **14**, 249.
Sarks S. H. (1976) *Br. J. Ophthalmol.* **60**, 324.
Sorsby A. (1972) *Rep. Public Health Med. Subj. No.* 128. London, HMSO.
Sperduto R. D. and Seigel D. (1980) *Am. J. Ophthalmol.* **90**, 86.
WHO (1966) Blindness: World Health Organisation Epidemiological and Statistical Report 19, 433. Cited by Ghafour I. M. et al. (1983).

2. PATHOLOGY OF THE AGEING EYE

Ralph C. Eagle jun. and Myron Yanoff

Ageing of the eye reflects the composite effect of ageing on its constituent cells and extracellular tissue. Basic cytopathological mechanisms in the elderly eye include cellular death or proliferation, the degeneration or elaboration of extracellular matrix material, and accumulation of pigments, minerals and other substances intra- or extracellularly. Visual loss, in both elderly and young, results generally from either death or dysfunction of the photosensory system, or opacification of transparent ocular media.

CELLULAR DEATH

Ocular cells vary in their ability to proliferate. Some, like the corneal epithelium, divide continually throughout life, replacing older cells that are discarded. In contrast, postmitotic cells such as retinal neurones are incapable of replication, and their number is thought to decrease with advancing age (Adams and Victor, 1981). The gradual loss may reflect, in part, 'preprogrammed cellular senescence'. *In vitro,* and presumably *in vivo,* human cells have a limited replicative lifespan (Cristofalo and Stanulis-Praeger, 1982). The faltering replicative capacity of older cells is thought to result from an acquired inability to initiate DNA synthesis, caused by regulatory abnormalities, not from accumulated genetic damage (Cristofalo and Stanulis-Praeger, 1982). Cells also succumb to the continual stress of environmental factors, such as free radicals (Tappel, 1975; Robbins and Cotran, 1979). Bathed with light and oxygen, the metabolically active outer retina is fertile soil for the generation of these highly reactive molecules. Produced by oxygen interactions during oxidation-reduction reactions, or by electromagnetic radiation, or both, free radicals are thought to damage cells by peroxidizing polyunsaturated fatty acids in their membranes (Tappel, 1975; Robbins and Cotran, 1979). Free radical damage to photoreceptor outer segments is probably the initial step in the accumulation of lipofuscin pigment in the retinal pigment epithelium (RPE) (Feeney, 1978). Genetic factors, i.e. the array of biochemical machinery encoded in each cell's inherited complement of DNA, also are important in the

8

response of cells to environmental stress. The stigmata of ageing may develop prematurely if cells harbour dysfunctional enzymes (e.g. the development of presenile cataract in galactokinase deficient individuals (Prchal, Conrad and Skalka, 1978)).

Under pathological conditions, major alterations in the cellular environment, e.g. profound retinal ischaemia secondary to central retinal artery occlusion, lead promptly to massive cellular death or dysfunction. The cells of a complex organ like the eye are highly interdependent. For example, the energy-intensive photoreceptors of the avascular outer retina are totally dependent on the RPE and inner choroid. Photoreceptor degeneration rapidly ensues when detachment of the retina anatomically precludes normal cellular interaction (Kroll and Machemer, 1968; Aaberg and Machemer, 1982). Fragile, postmitotic neurones also die when homeostatic mechanisms fail to maintain the intra-ocular environment within a relatively narrow physiological range. Glaucomatous retinal and optic atrophy is a striking example. Finally, cells may be killed by trauma. In the elderly, ocular trauma often is iatrogenic and surgical in nature.

THE PROLIFERATION OF CELLS

Non-neoplastic cellular proliferation is an important pathogenetic mechanism in ocular pathology. The presence of biochemical mediators or growth factors in their environment may induce normal cells to proliferate. Such substances are important in the proliferative reparative phase of inflammation. Hypothetical angiogenic factors produced by ischaemic retina are thought to stimulate ocular neovascularization (Henkind, 1978). Growth also may commence when suitable substrates or space for proliferation become newly available. Minor degenerative alterations in pristine ocular anatomy, e.g. posterior detachment of the vitreous, may provide *lebensraum* for cellular proliferation. This mechanism is operative in the formation of glial epiretinal membranes (Foos, 1980) (*Fig.* 2.1). In other instances, cellular proliferation results from a loss of normal cellular contact inhibition. Following cataract surgery, disease or atrophy of the corneal endothelium appears to facilitate surface epithelial invasion of the anterior chamber (epithelial downgrowth) (Yanoff and Cameron, 1977).

The increasing prevalence of neoplastic proliferation in the elderly reflects the progressive impotence of the immune surveillance system, as well as accumulated environmental damage.

THE EXTRACELLULAR MATRIX: ELABORATION AND DEGENERATION

The effects of ageing are obvious in the eye's extracellular tissues. When the ciliary processes of young and old eyes are compared, the latter

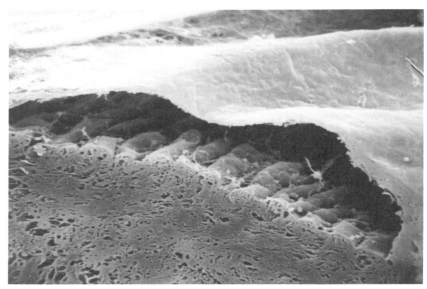

Fig. 2.1. Epiretinal glial membrane. Fibroglial sheet (above) is artifactitiously separated from inner surface of sectioned retina (below) revealing sinuously folded internal limiting membrane. SEM × 215.

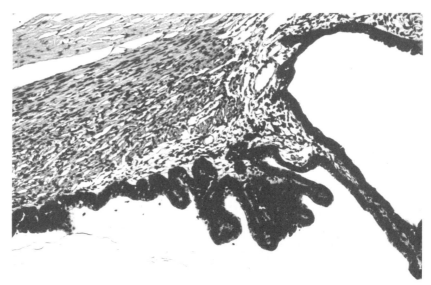

Fig. 2.2. Pars plicata, newborn eye. Delicate ciliary processes are composed only of central vascular core and enveloping ciliary epithelium. HE × 25.

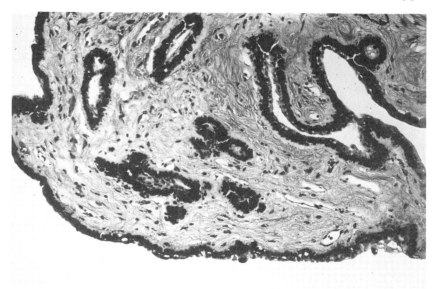

Fig. 2.3. Pars plicata, elderly eye. Blunting and hyalinization of ciliary processes reflects life-long accumulation of connective tissue in vascular core. (Compare with Fig. 2.2.) HE × 25.

appear thickened and white. Histopathologically, the 'hyalinization' reflects the life-long elaboration of collagen by vascular and ciliary epithelial cells (Figs. 2.2 and 2.3). Descemet's membrane and other ocular basement membranes (e.g. the inner cuticular portion of Bruch's membrane) thicken continuously throughout life. Under pathological circumstances excessive quantities of abnormal basement membrane material are produced by diseased or stressed cells. Important examples include cornea guttata, i.e. anvil-shaped posterior excrescences on Descemet's membrane produced by diseased endothelial cells in patients who have Fuchs' combined dystrophy (Yanoff and Fine, 1980; Waring et al., 1982) (Fig. 2.4), and retinal pigment epithelial drusen (Green and Key, 1977; Yanoff and Fine, 1982) and basal laminar deposits (Sarks, 1976) in senile macular degeneration (Fig. 2.5). In the exfoliation syndrome the fluffy white material seen clinically on the lens capsule (Fig. 2.6) and other ocular structures is probably abnormal extracellular matrix material secreted by epithelial cells throughout the anterior segment (Eagle et al., 1979; Dark and Streeten, 1982).

Degeneration of connective tissue in the eyelids is responsible for characteristic ageing changes, such as dermatochalasis (abnormally loose skin), orbital fat herniation, and senile entropion and ectropion. Histopathological examination of aged eyelid skin shows basophilia and

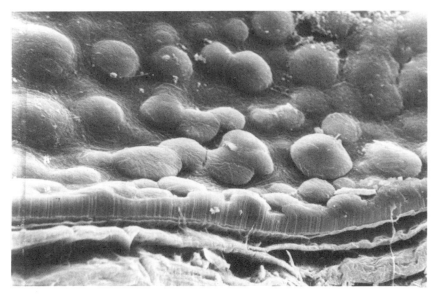

Fig. 2.4. Descemet's membrane, Fuchs' dystrophy. Multiple excrescences stud posterior surface of Descemet's membrane in a patient with advanced Fuchs' dystrophy. Cut surface of Descemet's membrane and posterior stromal lamellae are seen below. At left, endothelium is totally absent. SEM × 215. (Figure reproduced with permission from Yanoff and Fine's *Ocular Pathology: A Text and Atlas.* 2nd edition, Harper & Row, 1980.)

hyalinization of the dermis, fragmentation of collagen, and large quantities of elastic material insensitive to elastase digestion (Lund and Sommerville, 1957). This 'senile' or 'actinic' 'elastosis' may reflect, in part, abnormal production of elastic components (Austin et al., 1983). Degenerative ageing changes also are ubiquitous in the fibrous skeleton of the vitreous humour, the body's most delicate connective tissue. Extensive syneresis and posterior vitreous detachment are found in over 60 per cent of eyes in the 8th decade (Foos and Wheeler, 1982).

In the ageing eye the life-long accumulation and deposition of minerals, pigments and other substances, both within cells and extracellularly, become evident. Arcus senilis (gerontoxon), a characteristic stigma of age, results from the deposition of lipid in the peripheral cornea (and sclera where it is inapparent clinically) (Cogan and Kuwabara, 1959). Dystrophic calcification occurs in senile scleral plaques (Norn, 1974), in the degenerated cortex of advanced cataracts, and in Bruch's membrane where it is evident histopathologically as focal basophilia. Lipofuscin, a 'wear-and-tear' or ageing pigment, accumulates in the basal cytoplasm of the RPE (Streeten, 1961; Feeney-Burns et al.,

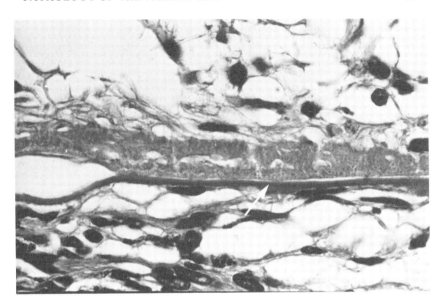

Fig. 2.5. Basal laminar deposit, senile macular degeneration. In this specimen, photoreceptors, retinal pigment epithelium and choriocapillaris are totally absent. Thick layer of basal laminar material is interposed between atrophic outer retina and inner surface of thickened Bruch's membrane (arrow). An area of artifactitious separation is seen at left. HE × 270.

1984). Most marked posteriorly, lipofuscin accumulation may be a factor in some cases of senile macular degeneration (Wing et al., 1978; Eagle, 1984).

OPACIFICATION OF THE OCULAR MEDIA

In the elderly corneal oedema caused by damaged or diseased endothelial cells is the primary cause of corneal opacification. In the adult, corneal endothelial cells do not usually proliferate or regenerate, and their number undergoes constant attrition with age (Mishima, 1982). When the endothelial population falls below a critical level, the 'endothelial pump' can no longer sustain the state of relative stromal dehydration compatible with transparency (Waring et al., 1982). In Fuchs' combined dystrophy (Yanoff and Fine, 1980; Waring et al., 1982) (*Fig.* 2.4) and in patients with the iridocorneal endothelial (ICE) syndrome (Eagle et al., 1979) oedema results from intrinsic endothelial disease. Most commonly, corneal decompensation reflects intra-operative endothelial trauma. 'Pseudophakic bullous keratopathy' following lens implantation now is a major indication for penetrating

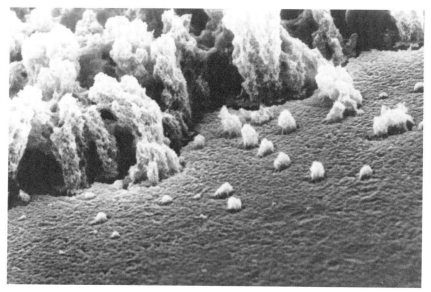

Fig. 2.6. Exfoliation syndrome, anterior lens capsule. Scanning electron microscopy reveals fibrillar nature of exfoliation material in peripheral granular zone. Artifactitious fissures near base of 'Busacca deposits' suggest deep involvement of underlying capsule. SEM × 840.

keratoplasty in the United States. In such cases of Fuchs' combined dystrophy microscopy (both light and electron) shows that guttata are buried by the subsequent proliferation of matrix material. Other cases show diffuse thickening and lamination of Descemet's membrane.

Histopathologically, an oedematous cornea shows loss of the normal artefactual interlamellar stromal clefts and a blurring or smudging of the collagen lamellae, which has been likened to 'cotton candy'. Subepithelial accumulation of fluid may lead to bullous keratopathy (*Fig.* 2.7). Fibroblasts beneath the epithelium elaborate a layer of connective tissue on the surface of Bowman's membrane, called a 'degenerative pannus'. In chronic cases epithelial abnormalities including reduplication, dyspolarity, intra-epithelial cyst formation, and elaboration of basement membrane material are common. Such changes are similar to those seen in map, dot and fingerprint dystrophy (Rodriguez et al., 1974). Patients with bullous keratopathy, which also may result from neglected glaucoma, are prone to acute infectious keratitis, corneal ulceration, and even perforation, often associated with secondary purulent endophthalmitis. The sudden decompression of a glaucomatous globe attendant on corneal perforation occasionally results in an expulsive choroidal haemorrhage (Winslow et al., 1974).

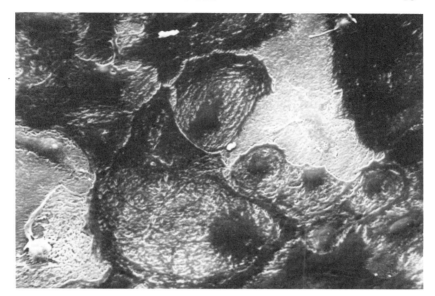

Fig. 2.7. Corneal endothelium, pseudophakic bullous keratopathy. Residual endothelial cells are pleomorphic and markedly enlarged. Descemet's membrane is partially denuded. SEM × 430.

Cataract, or opacification of the crystalline lens, is the ocular disease most synonymous with ageing. Histopathologically, three basic types of cataracts are recognized in elderly eyes: nuclear sclerosis, cortical opacification, and posterior subcapsular opacification (Yanoff, 1975; Klintworth and Garner, 1982). Nuclear sclerosis is an inevitable consequence of ageing inherent in the growth and development of the lens. A surface ectodermal derivative like the skin, the lens grows continuously throughout life. Although mature skin cells constantly are desquamated, older lens epithelial cells are inwardly sequestered and buried by the continuous accretion of new lens cytoplasm at the lens periphery. With increasing age the older cells in the nucleus degenerate and show increasing dehydration, dissolution of membranes, and loss of organelles. Ultraviolet light, which is absorbed primarily by the lens, may play an important role in this degenerative process (Klintworth and Garner, 1982). By light microscopy, a sclerotic nucleus appears increasingly homogeneous and eosinophilic, and lacks the normal artefactual clefts. Clinically and grossly, increasing amounts of yellow-brown urochrome pigment are evident. Progressive densification also increases the refractive index of the lens nucleus resulting in lenticular myopia that may temporarily obviate the need for presbyopic correction.

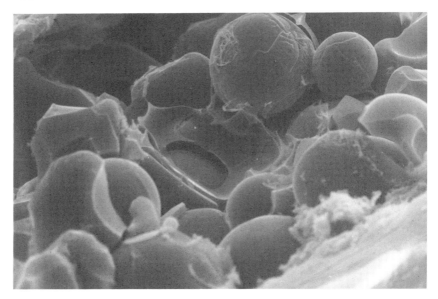

Fig. 2.8. Cortical cataract, Morgagnian degeneration. 'Water cleft' in cortical cataract contains Morgagnian globules which are of degenerated lens substance. SEM × 840.

Histopathologically, cortical ('soft') cataracts are characterized by fragmentation of lens fibres, clefts or spaces filled with eosinophilic spherules of degenerated protein called 'Morgagnian globules' (*Fig.* 2.8), or granular pools of liquefied cortex. Total liquefaction of the cortex is seen in Morgagnian cataract. As cortical degeneration progresses, the denatured lens substance exerts a considerable osmotic effect. Imbibition of aqueous produces a swollen, mature intumescent cataract that may precipitate lens-induced angle-closure glaucoma (*see* Chapter 8). Liquefied cortex also can leak though the intact lens capsule, stimulate a bland macrophage response, and occlude the trabecular meshwork (phacolytic glaucoma) (Flocks et al., 1955). Recent studies suggest that high molecular weight lens protein may play an important role in the production of this secondary open-angle glaucoma that usually responds to lens extraction and chamber lavage (Epstein et al., 1978). Hypermature cataract, a shrunken lens with a folded anterior capsule, results from increasing reabsorption of cortical material. Total spontaneous resorption of the lens is uncommon in the elderly, because the sclerotic nucleus resists dissolution. Iridescent intralenticular cholesterol crystals are common in cortical degeneration. Brilliantly birefringent crystals of calcium oxalate are usually confined to the sclerotic nucleus (Zimmerman and Johnson, 1958).

Posterior subcapsular cataract results from the migration of lens epithelial cells posterior to the equator of the lens. Abnormally situated beneath the posterior capsule, the cells form aberrant spherical lens fibres called 'bladder' or 'Wedl' cells. Located near the nodal point of the eye, a posterior subcapsular opacity tends to interfere with near vision early. Posterior subcapsular cataract tends to occur at an earlier age than cortical and nuclear cataracts and is commonly associated with concurrent ocular or systemic disease (e.g. retinitis pigmentosa (Eshagian et al., 1980) or diabetes mellitus), or exposure to toxins or drugs (e.g. systemic corticosteroids).

Although the classic clinical manifestations of the exfoliation syndrome (pseudoexfoliation of the lens capsule) are seen on the anterior surface of the lens, exfoliation material is probably produced by epithelia throughout the anterior segment (Eagle et al., 1979; Dark and Stretton 1982). Synthesized by lens epithelial cells, lenticular exfoliation is extruded through the lens capsule, forming 'Busacca deposits' that have been likened to magnetized iron filings (Ashton et al., 1965) (Fig. 2.6). Exfoliation material is also found on the ciliary processes, zonules, trabecular meshwork, and posterior iris, whose pigment epithelium shows a saw-tooth pattern of coalesced circumferential ridges. A form of secondary open-angle glaucoma called 'glaucoma capsulare' is the clinically most significant aspect of the exfoliation syndrome. True exfoliation or capsular delamination is not associated with glaucoma (Brodrick and Tate, 1979). Although classically associated with occupational exposure to infrared radiation, true exfoliation also occurs on a senile basis.

Although cataract surgery is successful in the vast majority of cases, early and late complications occur. The most devastating, though very rare, intra-operative complication is expulsive choroidal haemorrhage. As the globe is surgically decompressed rupture of a ciliary vessel produces a massive haemorrhage between choroid and retina that often expels the intra-ocular contents. Exogenous bacterial endophthalmitis usually presents 24–48 hours postoperatively with severe pain, injection, and hypopyon. Characterized by vitreous microabscesses, fungal infections are more indolent than bacterial infections in their course, and usually present 6–8 weeks following surgery. Other major postoperative complications include secondary glaucoma, aphakic bullous keratopathy, retinal detachment, and cystoid macular oedema.

The incidence of retinal detachment is quite high in aphakia (Jaffe, 1981). Although some cases follow surgical misadventure, the state of aphakia *per se* appears to predispose to rhegmatogenous retinal separation (retinal detachment with a tear). Aphakic retinal detachments typically result from small horseshoe tears at the posterior vitreous base (Eagle and Morse, 1976). Following intracapsular

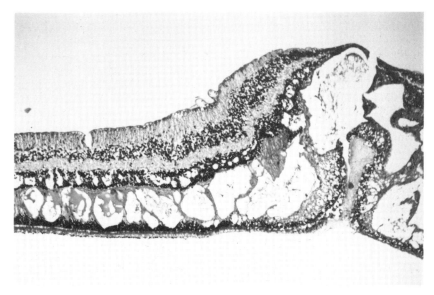

Fig. 2.9. Cystoid macular oedema. In specimen with chronic, endstage oedema, numerous cystoid spaces are present in outer plexiform layer. The retina is detached artifactitiously. HE × 15.

cataract extraction, increased mobility of the posterior face of the vitreous when detached predisposes to vitroretinal traction at this site. Retention of the posterior lens capsule in extracapsular extractions seems to lead to a lower incidence of retinal detachment.

Aphakic cystoid macular oedema (ACME, Gass and Norton, 1966) results from a breakdown in the blood-retinal barrier (Cunha-Vaz, 1979; Yanoff et al., 1984). Fluid that leaks from perifoveal capillaries collects in the retina in a petaloid pattern of radiating cysts centered on the floor of the fovea, best appreciated in the late stages of fluorescein angiography. Although spontaneously reversible in many cases, chronic ACME often leads to neuronal damage and permanent visual loss. In an electron microscopic study of several early angiographically documented cases, Fine and Brucker (1981) found massive intracytoplasmic oedema of Mueller cells and no extracellular fluid. Citing the important role of glial cells in the resolution of vasogenic cerebral oedema, Bellhorn (1984) has suggested that Mueller cell dysfunction may be an important factor in ACME. The cystoid spaces seen histopathologically in endstage cases (Tso, 1982) (*Fig.* 2.9) presumably result from the death of Mueller cells, if the stimulus for the condition is chronic (Fine and Brucker, 1981; Eagle, 1984). Clinical observations gleaned during the evolution of intra-ocular lens implantation suggest that inflammatory mediators produced in the anterior segment may be important in the pathogenesis of ACME (Miyake, 1978; Jaffe et al., 1982; Sears, 1984; Stark et al., 1984; Taylor et al., 1984; Yannuzi, 1984). An extremely high (10 per cent) incidence occurs in patients with intracapsular cataract extractions and iris-support intra-ocular lenses. A much lower (1 per cent) incidence is reported following planned extracapsular surgery and the implantation of posterior chamber intra-ocular lenses (Stark et al., 1984; Taylor et al., 1984). In the latter group, the posterior lens capsule limits contact between the vitreous, iris, and wound, and forms a barrier that impedes the posterior diffusion of prostaglandins and leukotrienes (Miyake, 1978; Sears, 1984; Yannuzi, 1984). The reputed therapeutic efficacy of prostaglandin inhibitors such as indomethacin also incriminates inflammatory factors (Minckler et al., 1975; Yannuzi, 1984) or, rarely, Whipple's disease should be suspected (Font et al., 1978).

DEATH OR DYSFUNCTION OF THE PHOTOSENSORY SYSTEM

In the elderly, glaucoma and senile macular degeneration (SMD) are the major cause of visual loss secondary to retinal or optic nerve damage (see Chapter 11).

The incidence of chronic open-angle glaucoma (COAG) (see Chapter 8), the most common type of glaucoma, increases with age. Although the pathogenesis of COAG is not understood, blockage of aqueous outflow is thought to occur in the general vicinity of the trabecular meshwork (Fine et al., 1981; Lee and Grierson, 1982). Abnormalities in endothelial 'giant vacuoles', deposition of glycosaminoglycans in the juxtacanalicular connective tissue, and impeded posterior uveoscleral outflow due to sclerosis in the region of the scleral spur are several pathogenetic hypotheses. An extensive, morphometric transmission electron microscopic study by Alvarado et al. (1984) has incriminated trabecular endothelial atrophy. Decreased trabecular porosity and compliance result from fusion and sclerosis of trabecular beams that have lost their endothelial covering. These endothelial changes resemble an exaggeration of the normal age-related decrease in trabecular endothelial density.

Acute closed-angle glaucoma also is most common in the elderly. The increasing size of the lens, which may be accelerated greatly by cataract formation, can compromise a previously unoccludable angle. Like phacolytic glaucoma, lens-induced angle-closure glaucoma usually occurs in the neglected cataractous eye of an elderly patient years after successful surgery in the fellow eye.

In SMD photoreceptor degeneration results from abnormalities in the RPE, Bruch's membrane, and inner choroid (Hogan, 1967; Lee, 1982;

Eagle, 1984). Throughout life, RPE cells gradually accumulate lipofuscin pigment and concurrently lose their apical melanin (Streeten, 1961; Feeney, 1978; Wing et al., 1978; Lee, 1982; Eagle, 1984; Feeney-Burns et al., 1984). These changes are most prominent posteriorly. Here, Bruch's membrane thickens and becomes increasingly PAS-positive and focally calcified. Transmission electron microscopy reveals that this thickening results from the accumulation of abnormal matrix material (Hogan, 1967; Hogan and Alvarado, 1967; Grindle and Marshall, 1978; Lee, 1982) or, possibly, from packets of damaged RPE cytoplasm (Burns and Feeney-Burns, 1980). Theoretically, the accumulation of this material in Bruch's membrane may interfere with the transport of metabolites and other substances between the choriocapillaris, RPE and outer retina (Grindle and Marshall, 1978). Excrescences of extracellular matrix material called 'drusen' are synthesized in the inner surface of Bruch's membrane by the RPE (Yanoff and Fine, 1982).

A disease spectrum, SMD is generally divided into atrophic ('dry') and exudative ('wet') forms on clinical grounds. Ophthalmoscopically, atrophic SMD is characterized by pigment clumping and rarefaction and progressive geographic atrophy of the RPE. In geographic RPE atrophy histopathology reveals loss of RPE, photoreceptors, and choriocapillaries (Green and Key, 1977; Eagle, 1984). Although the term 'choroidal sclerosis' has been applied to such lesions clinically, abnormalities of major choroidal vessels are not found (Howard and Wolf, 1964; Ferry et al., 1972; Sarks, 1973). Bordering atrophic lesions, the RPE cells are enlarged and contain excessive amounts of lipofuscin pigment (Weither and Fine, 1977; Eagle, 1984). It is unclear if this exaggerated ageing response has pathogenetic significance or is merely a nonspecific reaction. Large quantities of abnormal RPE lipofuscin have been incriminated in the pathogenesis of several atrophic macular dystrophies (Eagle et al., 1980; Frangieh et al., 1982; Weingeist et al., 1982). 'Hard' (cuticular) drusen, which are discrete, globular hyalin and intensely PAS-positive, are a characteristic feature in atrophic SMD (Sarks, 1980, 1982).

Exudative SMD is marked by the proliferation of subRPE neovascular membranes, exudation and haemorrhage. Disciform macular scars result from the organization and cicatrization of the haemorrhage. 'Soft' drusen, which appear confluent clinically and are difficult to distinguish from focal serous RPE detachments histologically, are typical (Sarks, 1980). A thick, continuous mantle of 'soft' basement membrane material called a 'basal laminar deposit' often is present on Bruch's membrane (Sarks, 1976) (*Fig.* 2.5). The material elevates the atrophic RPE and may provide the space or substrate for neovascular invasion (Eagle, 1984). In an elderly eye with RPE detachment, Green and Key (1977) demonstrated that the detachment occurred between the basal laminar deposit and the inner surface of Bruch's membrane. If detachment occurs where new vessels have invaded the basal laminar deposit, it is easy to conceive how subRPE haemorrhage could result.

Ischaemia *per se* probably is not a major factor in SMD. The retina's inner nuclear layer usually is preserved in SMD, but its outer part is atrophic in proven cases of choroidal ischaemia (Green and Key, 1977). Evidence suggests that loss of choriocapillaries in atrophic SMD is probably an involutionary phenomenon that follows photoreceptor and RPE death (Eagle, 1984).

Light may be an important contributory environmental factor in the development of SMD. SMD is relatively uncommon in blacks and other deeply pigmented individuals who have large amounts of uveal pigment (Wing et al., 1983). Hypothetically, the paucity of absorptive melanin in the choroid of blue-eyed, fair-haired people may subject their photoreceptors and RPE cells to a higher flux of photons back reflected from the sclera and choroid. The macula can be damaged by relatively brief exposures to high intensity light (Lanum, 1978). It does not appear unreasonable that 'normal' levels of ambient illumination could have deleterious effects over a lifetime.

TUMOURS OF THE EYE AND OCULAR ADNEXA

In the ophthalmic pathology laboratory the most frequent tumours, both benign and malignant, arise from sun-exposed eyelid skin. Squamous papillomas and seborrhoeic keratoses are common benign tumours in the elderly (Sassani and Yanoff, 1979). Basal cell carcinoma is the most common malignant eyelid tumour (Yanoff and Fine, 1982). Basal cell carcinomas occur most commonly on the lower lid, followed by upper lid, inner canthus and lateral canthus. Most commonly, the tumour afflicts white patients during the 7th decade. Although variable in clinical appearance, basal cell carcinomas classically are elevated nodules that have pearly margins and ulcerated surfaces. Incapable of metastasis, most are relatively 'benign' lesions that are cured by excisional biopsy. In the common nodular variant, histopathology typically reveals basophilic cords, islands, and fields of malignant basal cells that show peripheral palisading (*Fig.* 2.10). Between tumour lobules the intervening dermis undergoes a characteristic pseudo-sarcomatous change called 'desmoplasia'. The fibrosing or morphea-like type of basal cell carcinoma carries a more ominous prognosis than the nodular variant. In the morphea type the neoplastic cells proliferate as thin strands or cords that closely resemble the 'Indian-file' pattern seen in metastatic scirrhous breast carcinoma (*Fig.* 2.11). The morphea-like variant of basal cell carcinoma is aggressive and tends to invade underlying tissues deeply. Clinically, it is often difficult to delineate the

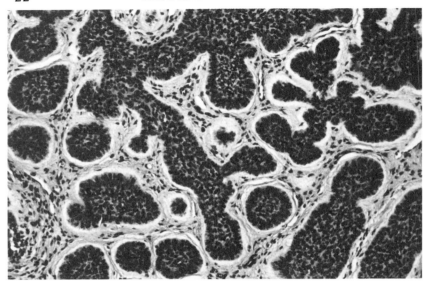

Fig. 2.10. Basal cell carcinoma, eyelid. 'Garden-variety' basal cell carcinoma is composed of cords and islands of basaloid cells with peripheral palisading surrounded by desmoplastic stroma. HE × 40.

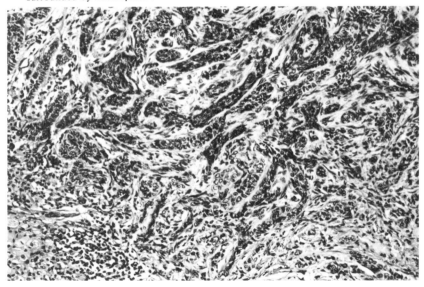

Fig. 2.11. Basal cell carcinoma, morphea-like variant. Cells of this aggressive form of basal cell carcinoma are arranged in slender tendrils that infiltrate deeper tissues. HE × 40.

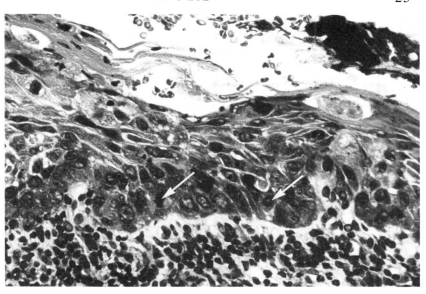

Fig. 2.12. Sebaceous carcinoma, pagetoid invasion. Epidermis of overlying eyelid skin has been invaded by malignant sebaceous cells with foamy cytoplasm. Arrows denote mitoses. HE × 270.

margin of a lesion without frozen section control. Neglected lesions called 'rodent ulcers' may destroy large portions of the face and can even cause death by central nervous system invasion. Squamous-cell carcinoma rarely involves the eyelids and occurs approximately 40 times less frequently than basal cell carcinoma (Kwitko et al., 1963; Yanoff and Fine, 1982).

Sebaceous carcinoma, the second most common malignant eyelid tumour, has a special predilection for the eyelids (Boniuk and Zimmerman, 1968; Rao et al., 1982). Clinically this tumour may mimic either the common benign inflammatory lesion chalazion or a diffuse blepharoconjunctivitis. Sebaceous carcinoma of the eyelid has an estimated 15 per cent 5-year mortality (Rao et al., 1982). Therefore recurrent chalazia should be submitted for histology, and atypical, recalcitrant blepharitis should be biopsied. Histologically, sebaceous carcinoma forms lobules somewhat reminiscent of normal sebaceous glands that lack peripheral palisading. In differentiated cases the tumour cytoplasm is foamy. In less differentiated cases, frozen sections stained for fat may reveal diagnostic intracytoplasmic lipid. An additional characteristic of sebaceous carcinoma is its propensity to invade and replace the overlying epidermis or conjunctival epithelium in a manner similar to Paget's disease of the breast (Russell et al., 1980) (*Fig.* 2.12).

The average age of patients with uveal malignant melanoma, the most common primary intra-ocular malignancy, is approximately 55 years. After 30, the incidence of this tumour rises steeply up to age 70. The tumour decreases in frequency after 80, and melanomas are very rare in patients over 80 (Paul et al., 1962). Patients over age 60 have a relatively poor prognosis despite enucleation (Westerveld–Brandon and Seeman, 1957). Although intra-ocular metastases are probably more frequent than primary tumours, many escape clinical detection in patients with terminal carcinomatosis (Bloch and Gartner, 1971).

VASCULAR DISEASE

In the elderly central retinal artery occlusion (CRAO) results commonly from cholesterol emboli (Hollenhorst plaques) or aggregates of fibrin and platelets shed from the surface of ulcerated carotid atheromata. Temporal (giant cell) arteritis can lead to bilateral CRAO and blindness if corticosteroid therapy is not promptly instituted. This chronic, inflammatory, usually granulomatous disease classically afflicts middle-aged or elderly women who have systemic symptoms; a presumptively diagnostic, markedly elevated erythrocyte sedimentation rate; and an enlarged, inflamed and pulseless superficial temporal artery (Keltner, 1982). Histologically, confirmatory temporal artery biopsy shows thickening and inflammation of the muscular media and adventitia, degeneration of muscle cells, and granulomatous inflammation centered on the fragmented internal elastic lamina (Albert et al., 1982).

Chronic open-angle glaucoma (Dryden, 1965) and retinal arteriolar sclerosis are important factors that contribute to central retinal vein occlusion (CRVO). In retinal arteriolar sclerosis, which is often a response to chronic hypertension, normally transparent vessels are thickened and opacified by an accumulation of fibrous tissue in their walls. Within a shared adventitial sheath, a sclerotic arteriole may precipitate venous occlusion (central or branch) by impinging on the neighbouring venule (Yanoff and Fine, 1982). Neovascularization of the iris develops in over 80 per cent of patients who have an ischaemic type of CRVO, but rarely in patients who have a nonischaemic type of CRVO (Priluck et al., 1980; Magargal et al., 1982; Yanoff and Fine, 1982; Yayreh, 1983). Optic nerve and retinal neovascularization are unusual clinical findings after CRVO. In branch retinal vein occlusion, however, optic nerve or retinal neovascularization, or both, may often occur (Yanoff and Fine, 1982).

ACKNOWLEDGEMENTS

Supported in part by the Gretel and Eugene Ormandy and Harry and Edith H. Hubschman Teaching and Research Funds, Scheie Eye Institute. Nestor G. Menocal and Dolores Ventura provided invaluable technical assistance. Photographic prints by Louise Pangborne. Word processing and manuscript by Deborah Nutter.

REFERENCES

Aaberg T. M. and Machemer R. (1982) In: Garner A. and Klintworth G. W. (eds) *Pathobiology of Ocular Disease.* New York, Marcel Dekker, p. 1351.

Adams R. D. and Victor M. (1981) *Principles of Neurology,* 2nd edition. New York, McGraw Hill, p. 419.

Albert D. M., Searl S. S. and Craft J. L. (1982) *Ophthalmology* **89**, 1111.

Alvarado J., Murphy C. and Juster R. (1984) *Ophthalmology* (In press).

Ashton N., Shakib M., Collyer et al. (1965) *Invest. Ophthalmol. Vis. Sci.* **4**, 141.

Austin P., Jakobiec F. A. and Iwamoto T. (1983) *Ophthalmology* **90**, 96.

Bellhorn R. W. (1984) In: Henkind P. (ed) *Cystoid macular edema. Survey Ophthalmol.* (Suppl) **28**.

Bloch R. S. and Gartner S. (1971) *Arch. Ophthalmol.* **85**, 673.

Boniuk M. and Zimmerman L. E. (1968) *Trans. Am. Acad. Ophthalmol. Otolaryngol.* **72**, 619.

Brodrick J. D. and Tate G. W. (1979) *Arch. Ophthalmol.* **97**, 1693.

Burns R. P. and Feeney-Burns L. (1980) *Trans. Ophthalmol. Soc. UK.* **78**, 206.

Cogan D. G. and Kuwabara T. (1959) *Arch. Ophthalmol.* **61**, 553.

Cristofalo V. J. and Stanulis-Praeger B. M. (1982) In: Karl Maramorosh (ed) *Advances in Cell Culture,* Vol II. New York, Academic Press, p. 1.

Cunha-Vaz J. G. (1979) *Survey Ophthalmol.* **23**, 279.

Dark A. J. and Streeten B. A. W. (1982) In: Garner A. and Klintworth G. K. (eds) *Pathobiology of Ocular Disease.* New York, Marcel Dekker, p. 1303.

Dryden R. M. (1965) *Arch. Ophthalmol.* **73**, 659.

Eagle R. C. (1984) *Ophthalmology* (in press).

Eagle R. C. and Morse P. H. (1976) *Ann. Ophthalmol.* **8**, 1072.

Eagle R. C., Font R. L. and Fine B. S. (1979) *Arch. Ophthalmol.* **97**, 510.

Eagle R. C., Font R. L., Yanoff M. et al. (1979) *Arch. Ophthalmol.* **97**, 2104.

Eagle R. C., Lucier A. C., Bernardino V. B. et al. (1980) *Ophthalmology* **87**, 1189.

Epstein D. L., Jedziniak J. A. and Grant W. M. (1978) *Invest. Ophthalmol. Vis. Sci.* **17**, 398.

Eshaghian J., Rafferty N. S. and Goossens W. (1980) *Arch. Ophthalmol.* **98**, 2227.

Feeney L. (1978) *Invest. Ophthalmol. Vis. Sci.* **17**, 583.

Feeney-Burns L., Hilderbrand E. S. and Eldridge S. (1984) *Invest. Ophthalmol. Vis. Sci.* **25**, 195.

Ferry A. P., Llovera I. and Shafer D. M. (1972) *Arch. Ophthalmol.* **88**, 39.

Fine B. S. and Brucker A. J. (1981) *Am. J. Ophthalmol.* **92**, 466.

Fine B. S., Yanoff M. and Stone R. A. (1981) *Am. J. Ophthalmol.* **91**, 91.

Flocks M., Littwinn C. S. and Zimmerman L. E. (1955) *Arch. Ophthalmol.* **54**, 37.

Font R. L., Rao N. A., Issarescu S. et al. (1978) *Arch. Ophthalmol.* **96**, 1431.

Foos R. Y. (1980) In: Nicholson D. H. (ed) *Ocular Pathology Update.* New York, Masson, p. 107.

Foos R. Y. and Wheeler M. C. (1982) *Ophthalmology* **89**, 102.

Frangieh T. T., Green W. R. and Engel H. M. (1982) *Arch. Ophthalmol.* **100**, 115.

Gass J. D. M. and Norton E. W. D. (1966) *Arch. Ophthalmol.* **76**, 646.

Green W. R. and Key S. N. (1977) *Trans. Am. Ophthalmol. Soc.* **75**, 180.

Grindle C. F. J. and Marshall J. (1978) *Trans. Ophthalmol. Soc. UK.* **98**, 172.

Hayreh S. S. (1983) *Ophthalmology* **90**, 458.

Henkind P. (1978) *Am. J. Ophthalmol.* **85**, 287.

Hogan M. J. (1967) *Trans. Ophthalmol. Soc. UK.* **87**, 113.
Hogan M. J. and Alvarado J. (1967) *Arch. Ophthalmol.* **77**, 410.
Howard G. M. and Wolf E. (1964) *Trans. Am. Acad. Ophthalmol. Otolaryngol.* **68**, 647.
Jaffe N., Clayman H. and Jaffe M. (1982) *Ophthalmology* **89**, 25.
Jaffe N. S. (1981) *Cataract Surgery and its Complications*, 3rd edition. St. Louis, CV Mosby, p. 576.
Keltner J. L. (1982) *Ophthalmology* **89**, 1101.
Klintworth G. K. and Garner A. (1982) In: Garner A. and Klintworth G. K. (ed) *The Pathobiology of Ocular Disease.* New York, Marcel Dekker, p. 1223.
Kroll H. J. and Machemer R. (1968) *Am. J. Ophthalmol.* **66**, 410.
Kwitko M. L., Boniuk M. and Zimmerman L. E. (1963) *Arch. Ophthalmol.* **69**, 693.
Lanum J. (1978) *Survey Ophthalmol.* **22**, 221.
Lee W. R. (1982) In: Garner A. and Klintworth G. K. (eds) *Pathobiology of Ocular Disease.* New York, Marcel Dekker, p. 1321.
Lee W. R. and Grierson I. (1982) In: Garner A. and Klintworth G. K. (eds) *Pathobiology of Ocular Disease.* New York, Marcel Dekker, p. 525.
Lund H. Z. and Somerville R. L. (1957) *Am. J. Clin. Pathol.* **27**, 183.
Margargal L. E., Donoso L. A. and Sanborn P. E. (1982) *Ophthalmology* **89**, 1241.
Minckler D. S., Font R. L. and Zimmerman L. E. (1975) *Am. J. Ophthalmol.* **80**, 433.
Mishima S. (1982) *Ophthalmology* **89**, 525.
Miyake K. (1978) *Jap. J. Ophthalmol.* **22**, 80.
Norn M. S. (1974) *Acta Ophthalmol. (Copenh)* **52**, 512.
Paul E. V., Parnell B. L. and Fraker M. (1962) *Int. Ophthalmol. Clin.* **2**, 387.
Prchal J. T., Conrad M. E. and Skalka H. W. (1978) *Lancet* **1**, 12.
Priluck I. A., Robertson D. M. and Hollenhorst R. W. (1980) *Am. J. Ophthalmol.* **90**, 190.
Rao N. A., Hidayat A. A., McLean I. W. et al. (1982) *Hum. Pathol.* **13**, 113.
Robbins S. L. and Cotran R. S. (1979) *Pathologic Basis of Disease.* Philadelphia, Saunders, p. 32.
Rodriguez M. M., Fine B. S., Laibson P. R. et al. (1974) *Arch. Ophthalmol.* **92**, 475.
Russell W. G., Page D. L., Hough A. J. et al. (1980) *Am. J. Clin. Pathol.* **73**, 504.
Sarks S. H. (1973) *Br. J. Ophthalmol.* **57**, 98.
Sarks S. H. (1976) *Br. J. Ophthalmol.* **60**, 324.
Sarks S. H. (1980) *Aust. J. Ophthalmol.* **8**, 117.
Sarks S. H. (1982) *Aust. J. Ophthalmol.* **10**, 91.
Sassani J. W. and Yanoff M. (1979) *Am. J. Ophthalmol.* **87**, 810.
Sears M. L. (1984) In: Henkind P. (ed) *Cystoid macular edema. Survey Ophthalmol.* (Suppl) **28**.
Stark W. J., Maumennee A. E., Sagadau W. et al. (1984) In: Henkind P. (ed) *Cystoid macular edema. Survey Ophthalmol.* (Suppl) **28**.
Streeten B. W. (1961) *Arch Ophthalmol.* **66**, 391.
Tappel A. L. (1975) In: Trump B. F. and Arstila A. U. (eds) *Pathobiology of cell membranes.* New York, Academic Press, p. 145.
Taylor D. M., Sachs S. W. and Stern A. L. (1984) In: Henkind P. (ed) *Cystoid macular edema. Survey Ophthalmol.* (Suppl) **28**.
Tso M. O. M. (1982) *Ophthalmology* **89**, 902.
Waring G. O., Bourne W. M., Edelhauser H. F. et al. (1982) *Ophthalmology* **89**, 531.
Weingeist T. A., Kobrin J. L. and Watzke R. C. (1982) *Arch. Ophthalmol.* **100**, 1108.
Weiter J. J. and Fine B. S. (1977) *Am. J. Ophthalmol.* **83**, 741.
Westerveld–Brandon E. R. and Zeeman W. P. C. (1957) *Ophthalmologica* **134**, 20

Wing G. L., Blanchard G. C. and Weiter J. J. (1978) *Invest. Ophthalmol. Vis. Sci.* **17**, 601.

Wing G. L., Weiter J. J., Delori F. C. et al. (1983) *Invest. Ophthalmol. Vis. Sci.* (Suppl) **24**, 170.

Winslow R. L., Stevenson W. and Yanoff M. (1974) *Arch Ophthalmol.* **92**, 33.

Yannuzi L. A. (1984) In: Henkind P. (ed) *Cystoid macular edema. Survey Ophthalmol.* (Suppl) **28**.

Yanoff M. (1975) In: Bellows J. G. (ed) *Cataract and Abnormalities of the Lens.* New York, Grune & Stratton, p. 155.

Yanoff M. and Cameron J. D. (1977) *Invest. Ophthalmol. Vis. Sci.* **16**, 269.

Yanoff M. and Fine B. S. (1980) *Ocular Pathology: A Text and Atlas.* Philadelphia, Harper & Row.

Yanoff M., Fine B. S., Brucker A. J. et al. (1984) *Survey Ophthalmol.* **28**, Suppl. 505.

Zimmerman L. E. and Johnson F. B. (1958) *Arch. Ophthalmol.* **60**, 372.

3. VISUAL CHANGES WITH AGE
Michael F. Marmor*

This chapter is concerned primarily with the quality of vision as a healthy person ages, rather than with the pathological changes of ageing. My purpose is two-fold: first, to provide a normal baseline on which to evaluate visual complaints in the elderly; second (and perhaps of greater importance) to provide an understanding of the visual needs and abilities of an elderly person.

PHYSICAL BASIS OF VISUAL AGEING
Changes in the Media and Optics of the Eye

Good vision depends upon the production of a focused image on the retina. Any decline in clarity of the media, or in the ability of the eye to focus, will limit visual acuity. For the most part, the cornea remains clear in old age, although the number of endothelial cells (which maintain clarity) diminishes so that the eye is more susceptible to corneal clouding after surgery or injury. The basic refractive power of the eye (i.e. near-sightedness or far-sightedness) remains relatively stable with age, except for changes that result from the ageing lens. The pupil becomes more and more miotic with age, producing effects which are partially off-setting: the small pupil (like a high f-stop on a camera) improves depth of focus, but at the same time lets in less light. The vitreous gel tends to condense and collapse with age; this process may cause floaters to appear, but these are rarely of visual significance. The major changes in the media occur in the lens, which becomes more dense, more yellow and less elastic with age (see Chapter 6). Frank clouding of the lens (i.e. cataract) is obviously pathological, but some degree of yellowing is present in virtually all older lenses. The aged lens adsorbs selectively the shorter wavelengths of light (blue colours) and tends to scatter light more than a young lens. These properties reduce the amount of light that reaches the

*Supported in part by National Eye Institute Grant EY01678 and the Medical Research Section of the Veterans Administration

28

retina, lead to altered colour sensitivity, and cause glare which interferes with the visual image.

Changes in the Neural Substrate of Vision

Once an image reaches the retina, the light must be transformed into neural signals, these signals must be coded for transmission by the optic nerve, and the brain must interpret the message for our conscious perception. Ageing causes a gradual loss of cells at all levels of this chain, from the photoreceptors to the visual cortex. For example, roughly 20 per cent of the photoreceptors are lost or damaged in a typical elderly eye. Fortunately, the visual system, like other organs in the body, has a degree of flexibility to allow for basic levels of function even in the presence of moderate cell loss and damage. This may explain why gross visual acuity can be surprisingly well-preserved in old age (although there will be deficits in subtle visual tasks that require fine tuning of the system).

The photoreceptors are exposed to radiant energy for a large portion of our lives, and such energy is potentially damaging to tissues. A mechanism must exist for renewing and recycling the light-absorbing photoreceptor outer segments. Skin grows continuously and sloughs the old cells; photoreceptors also grow continuously, but depend upon an adjacent cell layer, the retinal pigment epithelium, to phagocytose outdated membrane material and dispose of it by enzymatic digestion. Some of the waste products are indigestible and these contribute to the accumulation, with age, of lipofuscin. Progressive damage to the pigment epithelium is one cause of senile macular degeneration, which is dealt with elsewhere. Even in healthy aged eyes, the pigment epithelium loses much of its light-absorbing melanin pigmentation over the years.

The retina is embryonically a part of the brain, and is protected from proteins in the bloodstream by the blood-brain barrier. In the eye, this barrier is defined by tight junctions between cells of the intrinsic retinal capillaries and between cells of the retinal pigment epithelium. Loss of these barriers from ageing or vascular disease allows protein, fluid, and sometimes even blood vessels to enter the retina, with a resultant disruption of normal architecture and function.

One purpose in summarizing these physical changes is to emphasize that ageing in the eye is a multifactorial process. A person with better-than-average neurones but bad systemic vascular disease is as much at risk to lose vision as someone with healthy arteries but worse-than average loss of photoreceptors or damage to the pigment epithelium. We often cannot tell whether the visual changes in an elderly person are a result of suprathreshold damage to one critical element of the system, or of a cumulation of borderline damage to many elements.

Table 3.1. Distribution of individuals by age and corrected visual acuity in the better eye. Data from the Framingham Eye Study (Kahn et al., 1977)

Age group	20/25 (6/9) or better	20/40 (6/12) or better
52–64	98·4%	99·3%
65–74	91·9%	97·5%
75–85	69·1%	87·0%

VISUAL CHANGES WITH AGE

Presbyopia

Associated with the loss of lens elasticity is a gradual decline in the focusing power (accommodation) of the eye, up to age 55–60 when the process stabilizes. A child can keep a finger in focus nearly up to the nose, but this 'near point' recedes as we get older. By age 45–50 the near point has moved out to arm's length, which makes reading more difficult, and we call the eye 'presbyopic'. The small pupil of old age helps a little with depth of field, but not enough to compensate for the severe loss of focusing power. It is important to understand that the receding focus of presbyopia is not the same as 'far-sightedness' in a young person. The basic need for glasses (i.e. to see distant objects clearly) rarely changes after the mid-twenties. Presbyopia is simply a loss of focusing power that affects everyone, near-sighted or far-sighted, and necessitates an additional lens to see things close. Although presbyopia may be a nuisance, it is not a major health problem, because optical correction is so easily available.

Visual Acuity

The most prevalent measure of visual function, popularly and ophthalmologically, is 'visual acuity', which refers to the ability of the eye to resolve small objects under ideal conditions of brightness and contrast. Resolving power is unquestionably of importance to us, since it determines our ability to read fine print and recognize small objects at a distance. However, acuity measures only one limited parameter of vision; the real world rarely presents us with black letters on a white chart in a dark room.

In the recent Framingham survey, which was based upon prospective examination of the entire town of Framingham, Massachusetts, visual acuity was found to be remarkably well preserved in an elderly population (*Table* 3.1). Even over age 75, most individuals had better than 20/25 (6/9) acuity, and nearly 90 per cent had better than 20/40 (6/12), which is sufficient for driving and for reading ordinary fine print.

These data should not be interpreted to imply that visual loss is not still a serious public health problem. Over age 75, more than 10 per cent of the population had acuity poor enough to affect driving and other tasks, a figure which is hardly insignificant. Furthermore, both cataracts and senile macular degeneration are present in a sizeable fraction of the elderly population (*see* Chapter 1). Even when these disorders do not seriously affect acuity, they may impair other aspects of visual perception. Overall, these data tell us that complaints of poor or changing acuity by an elderly person should be taken seriously, and the excuse, 'he's old and shouldn't be seeing so well anyway,' is indefensible.

Finally, can we explain why visual acuity diminishes with age? Two general mechanisms seem to be involved. First, acuity is adversely affected by the various optical and media changes. For example, the smaller pupil of an elderly eye may degrade the image by diffraction; the aged lens is more dense than a youthful one, and may diffuse light and cause glare. Second, acuity will be affected by neuronal changes. Even if optical factors are compensated for experimentally, acuity is diminished in many older subjects. Weale (1982) has argued that this correlates with the dropout of cellular elements in the retina and higher visual pathways.

Contrast Sensitivity and Spatial Perception

Recognition of objects is rarely a matter of visual acuity alone. We do not judge a face, perceive texture, or choose where to step solely on the basis of minimally resolvable lines; we use a variety of other cues as well, including colour, pattern and contrast. The latter is of particular importance, and probably lies at the basis of many of our more complex perceptual functions. The neural circuitry of our retina and brain is, in fact, specifically designed to detect contrast. The photoreceptors recognize the presence of light; the next few layers of neurones respond rather poorly to diffuse light and are best stimulated by a sharp edge between light and dark. In essence, we recognize objects by their borders rather than by flat-coloured central areas: we perceive a green lawn by noting that it is green at the edges, and 'assuming' that the centre is also green since there are no borders to tell us otherwise.

Contrast sensitivity depends upon the spatial presentation of stimuli, as well as their differential brightness. Very thick objects or lines (i.e. targets having low spatial frequency) or very fine ones (of high spatial frequency) require higher contrast to distinguish than medium-size targets. Visual acuity, as measured clinically, is actually a special case of measuring contrast sensitivity at high contrast and vanishingly high frequency.

Contrast sensitivity remains relatively stable through middle age, but elderly individuals typically show a mild but definite loss of high and middle frequency contrast detection. Much of this loss may be explained by the decreased light entering the elderly eye and by light scattering in the older lens. Although a decrease in contrast sensitivity may seem subtle, it can be a major cause of visual difficulty: patients will complain that they can read the doctor's eye chart, but in the real world they just can't see as well as they used to, especially in dim light or under glaring lights. The point of consequence to the physician is that visual complaints and disability may be real even in the face of nominally normal visual acuity. Furthermore, depending on the contributing factors (pupil, lens, loss of neural connections, etc.), treatment may be possible by medical means or by modification of the visual environment.

Pattern and form perception are related visual functions which rely upon contrast detection to perceive the outline of an object, and cerebral factors to 'recognize' it. Elderly people are in general somewhat slower and less accurate in tests of pattern or form recognition, but the relative contributions of ocular vs cerebral pathology in causing this result have not been determined.

Adaptation

Sensitivity to light, and the ability to recover from changes in illumination, may both be diminished in older individuals. Much of this loss of sensitivity may be accounted for by the smaller pupil of old age (which lets in only about 30 per cent as much light) and by the increased density of the media (especially the lens) in the older eye; there is debate whether some of this intrinsic change in sensitivity may also have a neural basis. Older individuals typically require more time to recover from a bright light or flash that is temporarily dazzling. This can be a real problem in situations like night driving: oncoming headlights present a significant hazard if acuity is not quickly recovered. The cause of delayed recovery to photostress is probably a combination of factors. Media effects such as light scattering by the older lens will increase the amount of glare, and there may be neuronal loss or subclinical macular degeneration which impairs the timing of information processing.

Colour Vision

Gradual yellowing of the lens occurs with age, and as a result blue light is absorbed and scattered selectively, while the yellow and red end of the spectrum pass relatively unimpeded. Thus, blues become darker and less vivid, and there is a perceptual increase in warm tones. In aphakic individuals, no shift in colour sensitivity has been demonstrated with age. The degree of colour bias which occurs with age is quite variable, since lens changes vary considerably from individual to individual. Many older people have minimal yellowing, but individuals whose lenses are becoming brunescent, i.e. yellowish-brown, will show a very strong shift in colour sensitivity. Individuals with cloudy white cataracts may suffer a fading of colour vision, as contrast sensitivity is lost for colours as well as for light and dark, but they will not show much shift in spectral sensitivity.

Temporal Factors

Many aspects of vision relate to temporal phenomena, such as our ability to perceive flicker or to recognize images that flash by or follow closely one after another. Most of the temporal parameters which have been studied show a degree of failure with age, suggesting that, for whatever reason, the older individual is somewhat less able to follow and discriminate moving or sequential targets. This is another way in which the older individual may be at some visual disadvantage even though nominal acuity remains good. For example, driving requires the visual discrimination of moving objects more than static ones, and the elderly individual suffers a reduction in motion acuity. Losses of temporal resolution may arise from changes in the media, which decrease contrast sensitivity, but also from the intrinsic loss of neurones or other ageing changes in the visual circuitry.

ENVIRONMENTAL CONCERNS

In the absence of ocular disease, most elderly people have excellent vision under conditions of good illumination and high contrast. However, their vision may be marginal with respect to the more subtle components of perception, and will be very sensitive to changes in lighting, shading, viewing time, etc. The elderly person may require strong illumination to read, but at the same time will be unusually susceptible to glare from the light. Because blue light is scattered by the ageing lens, harsh fluorescent lighting is particularly bothersome to individuals with incipient cataracts. In general, warm incandescent lighting will be more comfortable and allow for better visual performance by older individuals. Interior design, labels, signs, etc., which use pastel shades and low contrast letters may be hard for the elderly to perceive, and these considerations should be taken into account when designing public facilities that will be used by older individuals.

Sympathetic counselling can help the elderly person adjust to these subtle visual limitations of age. Even if one is not an expert in geriatric ophthalmology or environmental lighting, common sense and a little inventiveness can go a long way. Lighting considerations, for example, rarely follow precise textbook recommendations. Rather, older individuals should be encouraged to experiment with different types of lamps and bulbs to find the combination which gives the highest contrast with the least interference from glare. Many common items, such as telephones, playing cards and books, are available in models that are designed with large or bright lettering for easy recognition. These high visibility products can simplify and speed up daily life even for older people who do not, strictly speaking, suffer low vision. Awareness of the functional limitations caused by limited contrast sensitivity, suscepti- bility to glare, reduced motion acuity, etc., can help the physician to advise a patient about walking, driving and other necessary activities. Finally, by being sensitive to these concerns, the physician can better judge when more active therapeutic measures such as cataract surgery would be justified. Cataracts rarely need to be removed for medical reasons; the primary indication is visual disability, and the level of acuity at which this occurs will depend upon individual activity and life style.

VISUAL CHANGES IN OCULAR DISEASE OF THE ELDERLY

There is often a fine line between ageing and disease. For example, when does senile yellowing of the lens become a cataract, or when does pigmentary atrophy in the macula become senile macular degeneration? In general, natural changes may be considered as acceptable sequelae of ageing until they interfere with ordinary levels of function. Older people are also at higher risk of development of certain diseases such as glaucoma, retinal detachment, vascular disease of the eye and diabetes. Some of these disorders induce specific visual disabilities of which the physician should be aware to distinguish them from 'normal' ageing.

We have already noted that a developing cataract not only reduces acuity, but causes difficulty with glare and reduced contrast sensitivity. Occasionally the distraction and frustration from scattered light and glare will warrant cataract surgery, even though visual acuity is not yet too severely impaired. Removal of the lens produces aphakia, a condition which has its own optical and visual problems. Correction with a fixed spectacle lens produces magnification, distortion of objects and a circular blind spot that may be very troublesome to an active person. Most of these symptoms can be avoided by the use of a contact lens or an implanted intra-ocular lens, both of which options are used increasingly by cataract surgeons. The removal of a densely yellowed lens may produce a sudden change in colour perception, particularly an increase in the brilliance and density of blues. Some sensitive individuals will be disturbed by this change or will notice conflict between the two eyes when only one cataract has been removed. The aphakic eye, having lost a short wavelength absorbing filter (the lens), may actually be sensitive to light in the near ultraviolet. These shorter wavelengths are potentially damaging to the retina at high intensities, and there may be wisdom in having aphakic individuals use an intra-ocular lens, contact lens, or spectacle made out of a material which absorbs wavelengths below 400 nm.

Open-angle glaucoma is a prevalent disease of the elderly which is particularly insidious because side vision is lost painlessly, and without the subject's awareness, until severe constriction of the visual field had occurred. Such 'tunnel vision' can be very disabling because an individual may see 20/60 (6/6) straight ahead but miss obstacles on the floor and to the side and thus have great difficulty walking in an unfamiliar environment. Unfortunately, there are no good optical aids for correcting visual field constriction.

Senile macular degeneration causes obvious disability when central acuity drops below levels which are comfortable for reading or driving. Fortunately, side vision and general mobility remain good. Severe macular degeneration, with its resultant loss of acuity, will obviously force a major adjustment in a patient's lifestyle; however, even milder degrees of macular degeneration can be very troublesome because acuity is not the only aspect of vision affected. Disruption of the macula causes poor contrast perception, heightened sensitivity to glare, delayed recovery from photostress, and poor temporal resolution. Sympathetic understanding, and attention to environmental factors, can help ease the adjustment to this condition.

Vascular disease and diabetes are relatively prevalent in an older population and will cause visual changes in proportion to the degree of ischaemia, haemorrhage, embolization, or proliferative change. Retinal detachment becomes more prevalent with increasing age, and there is an especially high risk in individuals who have had cataract surgery. The visual loss from detachment is directly related to the area of retina which has become separated. As might be expected, the photoreceptors gradually degenerate when separated from the choroid, and thus the likelihood of regaining good vision goes down with each week that a detachment remains unrepaired.

SUMMARY AND CONCLUSIONS

Many structures in the eye are affected by age, but of greatest relevance to vision are the lens (which becomes more dense, more yellow and less elastic) and the retina (which shows a gradual loss of neurones). Our range of accommodation (i.e. focusing) decreases gradually with age, but the reading problem that this causes is easily corrected by glasses. Visual acuity is not necessarily reduced in old age; in fact, the great majority of elderly people will maintain excellent reading vision. However, there is a gradual weakening of more subtle visual functions, such as the ability to distinguish contrast, to recognize forms and colours, to distinguish flickering lights, to recover from dazzle, etc. These difficulties may alter the subjective quality of vision, even while acuity remains normal.

Furthermore, these difficulties may be accentuated when ageing blends into pathology and the patient develops a symptomatic cataract or senile macular degeneration. Specific types of visual loss occur in disease of the older eye such as glaucoma, vascular disease and retinal detachment.

These data suggest that most older individuals retain good acuity, but have lost some of the subjective quality of their vision. Visual complaints beyond this baseline should be taken seriously, even in an elderly patient, because treatable pathology may be present. Understanding the subjective difficulties that elderly people have with vision helps the physician to provide reassurance and to offer positive suggestions to improve visual performance.

REFERENCES

Kahn H. A., Leibowitz H. M., Ganley J. P., et al. (1977) *Am. J. Epidemiol.* **106**, 17.

Weale R. A. (1982) *A Biography of the Eye.* London, H. K. Lewis.

FURTHER READING

Marmor M. F. (1982) In: Sekuler R., Kline D. and Dismukes K. (ed) *Aging and Human Visual Function.* New York, Alan R. Liss, pp. 59.

Marmor M. F. (1981) In: Ebaugh F. G., Jr. (ed) *Geriatrics for the Primary Care Physician.* Menlo Park, Addison–Wesley, p. 17.

Sekuler R., Kline D. and Dismukes K. (eds) (1982) *Aging and Human Visual Function.* New York, Alan R. Liss.

4. EXAMINATION OF THE EYE IN THE ELDERLY
I. G. Rennie and S. I. Davidson

HISTORY

Taking an accurate history from an older patient with an ocular problem is often difficult. All too often the elderly patient, who until recently has had excellent vision, will attribute failing vision to an inadequacy of her spectacles rather than of her eyes. Despite the problems, it is essential that the clinician establish at the onset of the consultation the precise nature of the patient's symptoms. Once the principal symptom or symptoms have been established, their duration and mode of onset should be ascertained. It is extremely important to note whether the problem affects one or both eyes.

Once the problem has been defined, the clinician should enquire if there has been any previous eye disease. If the patient wears glasses, the age when they were first acquired should be noted. Previous ocular trauma or surgery must be excluded. The clinician should always enquire if the vision in both eyes has always been equally good. It is easy to forget the fact that an eye which is amblyopic in childhood will still be amblyopic when the patient is elderly, and this may be important when cataract surgery is being considered. The documentation of a weak or lazy eye at this stage will often save both the clinician and patient unnecessary investigations later.

The clinician should then enquire into the state of the patient's general health. Particular attention should be paid to the presence of diabetes, hypertension, vascular occlusive disease, and arthritis. Any serious illnesses in the past should be noted. An accurate and complete drug history is essential. The clinician should not only note the drugs the patient is taking at present, but also any consumed in the recent past, and should always be alert to the possible ocular side effects of these drugs. Occasionally the patient's ocular problem may be entirely attributable to the ingestion of a particular drug. In this context the consumption of alcohol and tobacco should be noted.

37

EXAMINATION

Visual Acuity

An accurate assessment of the visual acuity must be obtained at the onset of the examination. If possible, both distance vision and near (reading) acuity should be evaluated.

The most popular method in Europe of assessing distance vision is the Snellen chart. The patient is seated 6 metres from the chart. One eye is then covered with an occluder. The patient is then asked to read the letters on the chart. The lowest (smallest) line accurately read by the patient is recorded. The procedure is then repeated with the other eye covered. If the patient normally wears distance glasses, they should be worn during the test. However, it is important to make sure that the patient uses distance glasses and not reading glasses for the examination. All too frequently the patient, when instructed to put glasses on and read the chart, will misinterpret the request, and attempt to use reading glasses with disastrous results. This error can be avoided if the patient is carefully instructed to use distance or 'going-out-in' glasses.

The patient who fails to read the letters on the chart adequately should be subjected to the pin-hole test. This procedure entails placing an occluder with a pinhole at its centre, on the visual axis, in front of the eye. This functions in a similar manner to the pin-hole camera and will improve the patient's ability to read the chart if the poor visual acuity is due to a refractive error rather than an organic cause. Whilst this test is occasionally useful, the elderly patient is often either physically or mentally incapable of performing this test. Furthermore, in patients with axial lens opacities, the use of the pinhole may significantly impair vision. There is no substitute for an accurate refraction in the elderly patient with poor vision. Occasionally the testing discloses a problem other than one of poor acuity. The patient with an homonymous hemianopia will often only read the letters down one half of the chart. The patient with visual agnosia will be unable to read the chart because higher cerebral function is impaired.

Reading vision may be evaluated using a near vision chart. Charts approved by the Faculty of Ophthalmologists may be used for this purpose (*Fig.* 4.1 *a* and *b*). Again the patient should be instructed to wear the appropriate glasses to accomplish this task.

Pupillary Reactions

Examination of the pupils is often cursory, with too much emphasis on stereotyped testing, and too little attention given to accurate observation. Careful assessment of the pupils and their reaction to stimuli can yield a wealth of information. A systematic approach is essential. The pupils should first be examined in normal ambient lighting. Any difference in size should be noted, as should be any irregularity in the shape of the pupils. The ambient lighting may then be reduced, but not extinguished, to facilitate the examination of the pupillary reaction to light. A bright light source should be employed for this purpose. It is better to stimulate one eye noting the direct light response, and then to stimulate the eye a second time, noting the reaction in the consensual eye, rather than trying to observe both reactions at once. If the patient is suspected of having an optic nerve or gross retinal disturbance, as for example after a retinal vascular occlusion, the afferent pupillary response may be elicited. This is accomplished by shining a bright light in one eye until the pupil is observed to constrict, and then 'swinging' the light source across to illuminate the other eye. The immediate reaction to the light in the second eye is observed. If its retina and optic nerve are functioning normally, its pupil will constrict when illuminated. However, if there is a defect in afferent transmission, the initial movement will be that of dilatation. Performed correctly, this test, in the absence of gross retinal pathology, provides a sensitive index of optic nerve function.

When the ambient illumination has been restored to normal the pupillary reactions in the synkinetic near reflex ('reaction to accommodation') can be evaluated. It should be noted that in the absence of any pupillary abnormality to light testing, testing of this reflex is unnecessary.

Ocular Movements

In the absence of suggestive symptoms such as diplopia, testing the ocular movements is probably unnecessary. If the ocular movements are tested it is as well to remember that both elevation and convergence may normally be diminished in the elderly.

EXTERNAL EXAMINATION

Periocular Tissues

Clinicians, when faced with an ocular problem, often fail to examine the periocular tissues adequately. Such omissions are unfortunate, for local dermatological or soft tissue disorders may affect the eyes. Giant cell arteritis is a not uncommon condition in the elderly; for this reason the temporal arteries should be palpated in any patient who complains of a sudden visual loss in one or both eyes. The skin and soft tissues around the eye should be carefully examined. It must be remembered that the skin around the eyes is a favoured site for the development of basal cell carcinomata. Attention should be paid to the medial canthi and adjacent tissues. Swellings in this region are often related to disorders of the nasolacrimal apparatus. Even in the absence of a swelling, gentle massage over the nasolacrimal sac will, not infrequently, produce regurgitation of its contents through the lacrimal puncta. It is particularly important to

TEST TYPES

N.5.

Now we have reached the trees—the beautiful trees! never so beautiful as to-day. Imagine the effect of a straight and regular double avenue of oaks, nearly a mile long, arching over-head, and closing into perspective like the roof and columns of a cathedral, every tree and branch encrusted with the bright and delicate congelation of hoar-frost, white and pure as snow, delicate and defined as carved ivory. How beautiful it is, how uniform, how various, how filling

— numerous renew assurance our sense ewe camera acorn assess cocoa source essence err —

N.6.

how satisfying to the eye and to the mind—above all, how melancholy! There is a thrilling awfulness, an intense feeling of simple power in that naked and colourless beauty which falls on the earth, like the thoughts of life—life pure and glorious and smiling—but still life. Sculpture has always the same effect on my imagination, and painting never. Colour is life.—We are now at the end of this magnificent avenue, and at the top of a steep eminence commanding

— ear race access cannon emu error mace summon season nevermore overawe crane —

N.8.

a wide view over four counties—a landscape of snow. A deep lane leads abruptly down the hill; a mere narrow cart-track, sinking between high banks clothed with fern and furze and low broom, crowned with luxuriant hedge-rows and famous for their summer smell of thyme.

— cam macaroon overseas race ocean excess nurse answer raven —

N.10.

How lovely these banks are now—the tall weeds and gorse fixed and stiffened in the hoar-frost, which fringes round the bright, prickly holly, the pendent foliage of the bramble, and the deep orange leaves of the pollard oaks ! Oh !

— accurse can name one recess oversee own newcomer —

N.12.

this is rime in its loveliest form ! And there is still a berry here and there on the holly, "blushing in its natural coral," through the delicate tracery, still a stray hip or haw for the birds, who

— same accrue car oxen recover ensnare nerve —

N.14.

abound here always. The poor birds, how tame they are, how sadly tame! There is the beautiful and rare crested

— ease on manner even crown cover arose —

N.18.

wren, "that shadow of a bird," as White, of Selbourne, calls it, perched in the middle

— severe room caravan era —

N.24.

of the hedge, nestling, as it were,

— surname seven arrow —

Fig. 4.1. Near visual acuity test chart.

N.36.

amongst the cold, bare
— occur reserve arc —

N.48.

boughs, seeking,
— ran overrun —

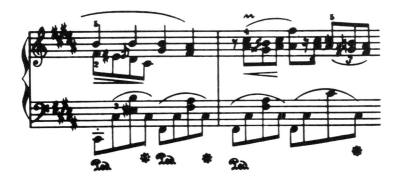

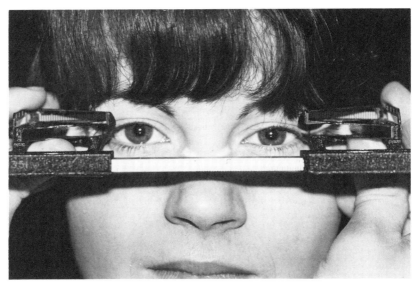

Fig. 4.2. A Hertel exophthalmometer.

exclude such a reservoir when a patient presents with a chronic unilateral conjunctivitis.

The position of the globes should be examined. Any proptosis, either unilateral or bilateral, should be carefully evaluated. A Hertel exophthalmometer (*Fig.* 4.2) is the most accurate method of quantitatively assessing degrees of proptosis. If one globe appears displaced, the orbital rim should be palpated. This will occasionally reveal the presence of an orbital mass such as a metastatic deposit.

Eyelids

The eylids are often the source of considerable problems in the elderly. Senile entropions and ectropions (*see* Chapter 5) are a common cause of discomfort and surprisingly they are often overlooked. It is important to exclude an entropion in any patient with a persistent foreign body sensation or with a chronic conjunctivitis. Entropions may be intermittent. If it is suspected, the clinician should instruct the patient to close the eyes tightly and then open them. The intermittent entropion may then be observed.

Severe forms of ectropion are usually obvious, the patient complaining of a persistent watering on the affected side. On examination a lax lower lid, in which the margin is no longer in apposition to the globe, is noted. Subtle degrees of ectropion occur, often affecting only the medial aspect of the lower lid. Again the patient complains of epiphora.

Misdirected eyelashes (trichiasis) commonly abrade the cornea of elderly individuals, producing a persistent foreign body sensation. Blepharitis, a low grade inflammation of the lid margin, produces crusting and scaling of the eyelashes. This condition may be associated with other ocular disorders, for example, kerato-conjunctivitis sicca (*see* Chapter 5). The relative positions of the upper lids should be inspected to exclude a ptosis. Normally, the upper lids cover the superior 2 mm of the cornea.

Cornea and Conjunctiva

Once the periocular tissues and eyelids have been inspected, attention may be turned to the globes. The examination should proceed in an orderly manner with external features, the conjunctiva, cornea, and anterior sclera being examined sequentially. Any focal or generalized hyperaemia of the conjunctiva should be examined. In this context, the term 'conjunctivitis' should be used with caution. Many clinicians use this to describe any red, inflamed eye. This is not only misleading, but occasionally dangerous. Conjunctivitis is a specific disease process in which the inflammation is restricted to the conjunctiva. Focal areas of hyperaemia should be viewed with suspicion, for conjunctivitis usually affects the entire conjunctival surface. If the patient complains of a foreign body sensation the upper lid should be everted and the tarsal surface examined for the presence of a foreign body.

The cornea is best examined with the aid of a bright light source. Ideally, of course, the illumination and magnification provided by slit-lamp biomicroscopy should be employed. When such facilities are not available, or the patient is not ambulant, the cornea may be examined with the aid of a loupe and pen torch. Staining of the cornea with a vital stain such as sodium fluorescein facilitates this examination. Areas of epithelial devitalization fluoresce brightly when a drop of fluorescein is administered to the conjunctival fornix. This effect is considerably enhanced by using a light source that emits cobalt blue light (*Plate I*). Pen torches incorporating the correct filter are available for this purpose.

Intra-ocular Pressure Measurement

The intra-ocular pressure should be measured in all elderly patients, whether or not the symptoms are referable to a glaucomatous problem. Digital palpation of the globe has no place in modern ophthalmic practice. To the inexperienced all globes tend to feel 'hard'. Even in experienced hands, palpation can only provide a crude guide to the intra-ocular pressure. If slit-lamp biomicroscopy is available, the Goldmann applanation tonometer (*Fig.* 4.3) provides the simplest and most accurate means of measurement of the intra-ocular pressure. Alternatively, the immobile patient can be assessed using a Perkins hand-held

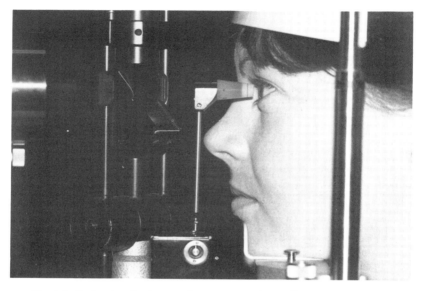

Fig. 4.3. Estimating the intra-ocular pressure using a Goldmann applanation tonometer in conjunction with a slit-lamp.

applanation tonometer (*see Fig.* 8.2). However, this is usually more difficult to use than its slit-lamp counterpart.

OPHTHALMOSCOPY

Examination of the ocular media and fundi are essential. Senile miosis is common, and will severely impair visualization of the fundus unless the pupil is dilated, which can be easily achieved using a short-acting mydriatic. The drug of choice is tropicamide 0·5 per cent, which has the advantage of brevity of action and minimal effect on accommodation. Fear of precipitating an attack of acute angle-closure glaucoma has led many clinicians to avoid dilating the pupil. In reality the risk with tropicamide is minimal. However, one should always warn the patient to return immediately if a red or painful eye develops within 24 hours of the examination. Attempted 'reversal' of the mydriatic with pilocarpine is practised by many but is ineffectual and potentially harmful. Diagnostic pupil dilatation should not be performed on patients suffering from any form of head injury, for this may deprive the clinician of an important parameter of their neurological status.

Before a detailed examination of the ocular fundus is made, the clinician should always examine the nature of the red reflex. Opacities in the ocular media, especially of the crystalline lens, will appear as defects in this reflex. Both the character and the relative density of a lens opacity can be evaluated using this simple technique. It is well to remember that if the clinician is unable to see into the eye, the patient will be unlikely to see out of it.

The examination of the ocular fundus should be carried out in a systematic manner. It is prudent to assess the optic disc at the start of the examination. The major vessels should be examined and traced to the periphery. The superior, inferior, and lateral quadrants should then be examined. Finally the macula should be evaluated. This latter procedure is of little value if the pupil has not been dilated. The occasional patient with a subtle or early maculopathy will require a stereoscopic fundal examination. This may be performed by an ophthalmologist using either a Hruby lens or contact lens in combination with a slit-lamp biomicroscope. These methods neutralize the refractive power of the cornea and permit visualization of the fundus.

EVALUATION OF RETINAL FUNCTION IN A PATIENT WITH OPAQUE OCULAR MEDIA

Elderly patients frequently present with an eye (or eyes) in which dense lens opacities make examination of the fundus impossible. In such patients it is desirable to assess their retinal and macular function. Several simple tests may be used.

Projection

The examiner occludes the patient's unaffected eye. A bright torch is then shone into the affected eye obliquely, from either the superior, inferior, nasal, or lateral quadrant. The patient is then asked to state or point to the origin of the light. This procedure is then repeated for the other quadrants. Failure to detect the light source from a quadrant or quadrants suggests a defect in retinal function. While this test may arouse suspicion, too much emphasis must not be placed upon it. The clinician must be aware that an extremely dense lens opacity may produce apparent projection defects. Conversely patients with a shallow retinal detachment may still be able to perceive the light accurately.

Macular Function

Senile macular degeneration and cataracts are common disorders in the elderly. Not surprisingly, the two conditions frequently occur together. Before submitting a patient with dense lenticular opacities to surgery, some attempt should be made to assess macular function.

The Maddox Rod test is simple to perform, providing the patient understands fully what is required. A Maddox Rod is a lens made of red

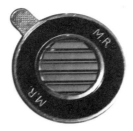

Fig. 4.4. A Maddox rod.

glass with one surface grooved to produce the effect of several parallel rows of double prisms (*Fig.* 4.4). When a light is shone through it a red linear streak at right angles to the grooves is observed. The test is performed by holding the lens close to the patient's eye and illuminating it with a torch. If the macula is normal the patient will perceive a continuous red line. If it is abnormal the patient will note a break in the centre of the line.

VISUAL FIELDS

Simple testing of the visual fields by the confrontation method may yield useful information, providing both the patient and examiner understand the nature of the test. In general, confrontation testing will only disclose gross defects in the visual fields, usually those of neurological origin. Attempting to elicit subtle scotomas by confrontation will fatigue both patient and examiner. The elderly patient often has poor attention, so that it is prudent to keep the test as simple as possible. One relatively simple method is the finger counting test. The patient is instructed to cover one eye with the palm of the hand, and look with the other eye at the tip of the examiner's nose. The examiner, having divided the patient's visual fields into four imaginary quadrants, positions his hands in two of the fields and raises one or two fingers on each hand. The patient is instructed to count the number of raised fingers whilst still looking at his nose. This should be repeated several times until all four quadrants have been repeatedly challenged. A field defect should be suspected if the patient repeatedly fails to report the correct number of fingers when one hand is placed in the same quadrant or quadrants. Any suspected field defect should always be confirmed by perimetry.

Central Field of Vision

Frequently a patient with a good or relatively good visual acuity will complain of distortion in central vision. The distortion may be a change

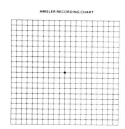

Fig. 4.5. Amsler grid, a quarter normal size.

in shape (metamorphopsia) or size (e.g. micropsia) of the image. In the elderly, this is usually due to senile macular degeneration. The Amsler grid (*Fig.* 4.5) is a simple method of assessing distortion of the central vision. The patient is instructed to look at the spot in the centre of the grid. With the unaffected eye occluded the patient is then asked if he notes any distortion of the horizontal or vertical lines. Often the patient will be able to mark on the chart the areas of distortion. Quite subtle defects in the central vision can be elicited by using this test.

5. COMMON EXTERNAL EYE DISEASES IN THE ELDERLY
John Williamson

This chapter deals with the diseases of the external eye most frequently observed in the elderly population. Diseases of the lacrimal and accessory lacrimal glands are considered first, and their close and confusing relationship with various connective tissue diseases is examined in detail. For the sake of continuity, and because their symptoms are often closely related and often confused with each other, lid abnormalities and tear drainage problems are then discussed.

CONJUNCTIVITIS

Conjunctivitis is common in all age groups. However, recurrent or persistent conjunctivitis in the elderly should alert the physician to the possibility of underlying lacrimal disease, faulty lid apposition, or defective tear drainage.

Keratoconjunctivitis Sicca (KCS)

In the normal population there is a steady increase in the incidence of the dry eye unrelated to connective tissue disease (CTD), from 2 per cent at 45 years up to 16 per cent at 80 years of age. When KCS is found in association with a CTD, the latter is usually rheumatoid arthritis (RA; over 60 per cent of all cases), and less often systemic lupus erythematosus, polymyositis, progressive systemic sclerosis or polyarteritis nodosa; the most recent term for this combination is 'secondary Sjögren's syndrome'. In the absence of CTD the term 'primary Sjögren's syndrome' or the 'sicca syndrome' has been used. KCS of the elderly is usually a form of primary Sjögren's syndrome. All these CTDs except rheumatoid arthritis are uncommon, and it is thus to be expected that in most elderly patients rheumatoid arthritis is the cause.

Since the incidence of KCS in secondary Sjögren's syndrome is only 10 per cent, it is clear that the largest number of patients with dry eyes are elderly, and do not suffer from a CTD. The dry eye thus is more commonly present in the elderly in the absence of any systemic autoimmune activity, and it is, in these patients, aetiologically and pathologically distinct from secondary Sjögren's syndrome and from other forms of primary Sjögren's syndrome.

Pathology: With advancing years there is a progressive atrophy of the lacrimal gland acini and ducts, probably preceded by minimal lymphocytic infiltration. 'Ageing' of the lacrimal and accessory lacrimal glands may be the result of repeated attacks of mild dacryocystitis. The mucopolysaccharide components of the glandular tissue are alkaline in healthy young adults, become neutral by middle age and are distinctly acidic in the elderly. In old age, even if there appears to be adequate lacrimal fluid-producing tissue, the product contains less lysozyme and lactoferrin components to combat infection. The conjunctiva also develops alternating patches of epithelial hyperplasia and dystrophy, with an overall reduction in the goblet cell content. In some instances all goblet cells have vanished.

In contrast, the lacrimal gland in secondary and most forms of primary Sjögren's syndrome shows intense lymphocytic infiltration, to the point of pseudo-follicle formation, followed by progressive destruction of the normal acinar epithelium and its replacement by acellular hyaline fibrous tissue. The conjunctival changes are also quite distinctive, and totally different from those in old age. Stratification of the conjunctiva, flattening and loss of the microvilli surface, superficial layer separation and dramatic reduction of the goblet cells are specific to both forms of Sjögren's syndrome.

Diagnosis: The cardinal features of dry eyes are a chronic gritty or sandy feeling, and less often itch in the eyes. Other less specific symptoms include tired eyes, dryness (rarely alluded to directly), excess ropey discharge, and photosensitivity. It is significant that most patients remain undiagnosed for years, receive an assortment of antibiotics, and buy a multitude of commercially prepared 'eye washes'. These treatments may work for a time since superimposed infection is frequent. Almost 30 per cent of undiagnosed KCS patients with secondary Sjögren's syndrome present with infected lash roots (blepharitis).

There is no simple certain sign of the dry eye. More often than not the eye appears perfectly normal to the casual observer. If the upper lid is rolled backwards and upwards with the thumb in a quick single movement, in 40 per cent of untreated patients with dry eyes there will be a small 'explosion'—a crackling noise. This only happens on the first occasion, and will not be repeatable for half an hour or so. It is due to the lack of lubrication between lid and eyeball. Look for blepharitis and observe ropey discharge in the lower fornices (*Fig.* 5.1. and *Plate II* 1). A lacklustre cornea may also be evident.

Schirmer's standardized filter test strips are placed in the lower fornices for 5 minutes while the patient is given 10 per cent ammonia to inhale. If a normal volume of lacrimal fluid is being produced, the strips should be wet to more than 15 mm at the end of this time. This is not a

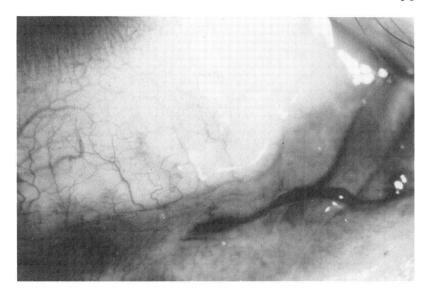

Fig. 5.1. Ropey discharge in lower fornix—typical of the very dry eye.

very reliable test, and errs on the side of over-diagnosis. At the geriatric out-patient clinic or the patient's bedside the dye Rose Bengal (which comes in individual single doses) can be instilled. A topical anaesthetic should always be to hand; benoxinate or amethocaine are suitable. In patients with a positive test the dye is usually irritant; this is a significant sign, and hence the need for topical anaesthesia. It is possible to see with a magnifying loupe, or even with the naked eye, the dark red stained mucous plaques and stringy discharge characteristic of the dry eye (*Fig.* 5.2).

Further identification requires biomicroscopic examination. In 80 per cent of patients the interpalpebral conjunctiva stains in a wedge-shaped area with its base towards the corneo-conjunctival junction. The pattern varies from fine punctate to coarse conglomerate patches (*Fig.* 5.3). In severe cases, the cornea is also involved with a similar variation in intensity of staining. Filaments of dye-stained mucus indicate particularly uncomfortable irritant areas.

In general, the dry eye of old age is less severe than that of Sjögren's syndrome. Staining with Rose Bengal is more often fine punctate than coarse and filamentous.

Management: Conscientious replacement of tears and constant vigilance against infection are the principles of management. Patients must be urged to use artificial tears at least four times daily and much

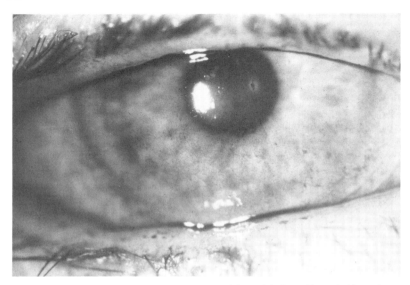

Fig. 5.2. A mixture of fine and coarse staining with Rose Bengal. Note the filamentous appearance in the pupillary area.

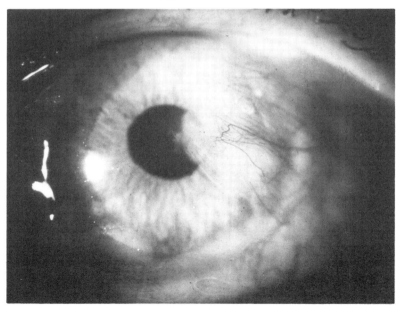

Fig. 5.3. Repeated corneal ulceration, vascularization, and pseudopterygium formation in a patient with KCS.

more often if symptoms persist. There are many suitable solutions available, most of which vary little in content from Barrie Jones' 6th Formula of a dilute alkaline solution of carboxymethyl cellulose. Examples are hypromellose 0·3 per cent, Liquifilm Tears, Tears Naturale, Isopto Alkaline, and Adapt. It is important that the container should be easily opened and the drops readily expressed, in view of the difficulties created by frail ageing hands. Several attempts have been made to produce reservoirs of artificial tears attached to spectacles (even power driven) but to date these have had limited success. When infection supervenes, topical antibiotics are required. When excessive ropey discharge persists the mucolytic agent acetylcystein 5 to 10 per cent is very effective; patients must be warned that these drops are somewhat irritant, though it is worth persisting for a month.

Patients with dry eyes are susceptible to warm, dry, and smoke-filled atmospheres. Direct radiation from electric fires is particularly drying, gas and coal less so. The patient should be advised to use humidifiers—at least a shallow plate topped up with water.

Complications: It is uncommon for the elderly patient with KCS alone to develop complications of the dry eye syndrome. On the other hand, the elderly patient with secondary Sjögren's syndrome is as likely to run into difficulties as the youngest rheumatoid patient. It is quite untrue to suggest that the ocular process in Sjögren's syndrome eventually burns itself out, leaving the patient asymptomatic.

Complications occur in less than 10 per cent of large series of patients with secondary Sjögren's syndrome. However, when they develop the results are particularly serious. Infection in KCS is common; apart from blepharitis, corneal ulceration due to bacterial or viral agents may occur (*Fig.* 5.4). Appropriate antibiotic or antiviral therapy is indicated (e.g. chloramphenicol or acyclovir). Progressive conjunctival and sub-conjunctival contracture can produce symblepharon (*Fig.* 5.5); pemphigoid should then be considered as a differential diagnosis. Corneal pannus formation may be sight-threatening, and perforation is very grave (*Plate II* 2). The management of all the last three complications is unsatisfactory. Severance of symblepharon may merely induce further contracture. There is no effective treatment for pannus. Perforating ulcers may perhaps heal but leave dense scars which do not respond to corneal grafting, since the same process of ulcerating and perforation always occurs in the grafted tissue.

Summary: The dry eye develops in up to 16 per cent of the elderly without connective tissue disease. In addition elderly rheumatoid patients have the usual 10 per cent incidence of Sjögren's syndrome. The disorders are aetiologically and pathologically distinct. However, the clinical presentations and management are the same. Vigorous application of artifical tears and vigilance for complicating infection are essential.

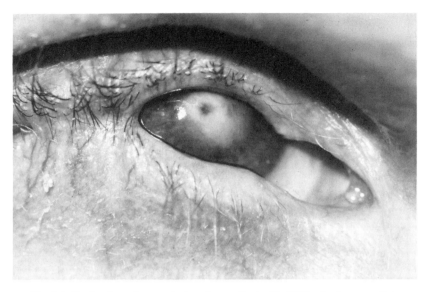

Fig. 5.4. Perforation of corneal ulcer in a patient with KCS who has a partial tarsorrhaphy.

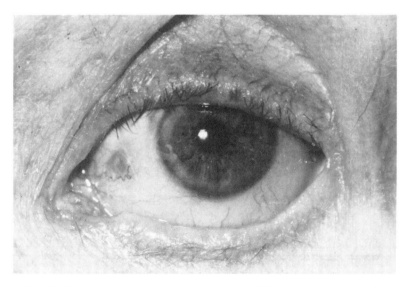

Fig. 5.5. Senile hyaline degeneration of the sclera. This appearance is typically situated close to the insertion of a rectus muscle.

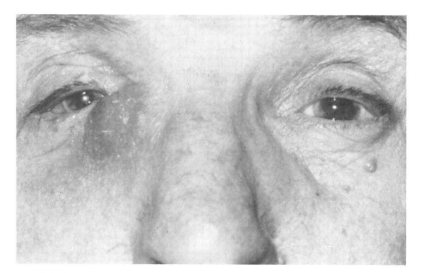

Fig. 5.6. Acute dacryocystitis.

SCLERITIS AND EPISCLERITIS

Scleritis—inflammation of the scleral tissues—occurs in 0·2 per 1000 of the population, and in 7 per 1000 of adult patients suffering from rheumatoid arthritis (RA). Conversely, 30 per cent of all scleritis patients suffer from RA; the remainder have no other disease, or occasionally one of a variety of CTD, such as Wegener's granulomatosis, polyarteritis nodosa, temporal arteritis, dermatomyositis, systemic lupus erythematosus, or ankylosing spondylitis. In addition, tuberculosis and sarcoidosis have been reported as the only other concomitant finding in scleritis. When the adjacent cornea is inflammed the term 'sclero--keratitis' is appropriate.

The above list of associated diseases suggests that the elderly are unlikely to be subject to the development of scleritis for the first time in old age. This is indeed the case; in the author's experience an attack of scleritis in a patient over 70 years of age is excessively rare, usually occurring where there is evidence of previous activity.

Episcleritis—inflammation of the episcleral tissues—is a mild, transitory, self-limiting disorder of no prognostic or diagnostic significance. Difficulty arises on occasion in differentiating it from scleritis, and it has been reported in the same range of patients as scleritis.

Pathology: In 90 per cent of cases there are no specific histological features of scleritis. However, recognizable rheumatoid nodules have been seen, and in tuberculosis and sarcoidosis at least part of the scleral inflammation may be characteristic of the parent disease.

Diagnosis: Scleritis nearly always affects the anterior segment of the eye and is easier to diagnose in natural rather than artificial light. In daylight conditions there is a characteristic mauve discoloration of the sclera. Prolonged bouts of intractable pain are usual, and there is no discharge.

There are several different phases of activity recognizable in scleritis. Nodules should hint at RA, if it is not already apparent (*Plate III* 1). Necrosis can present a terrifying picture which suggests that the globe will rupture. Fortunately this is rare; B-scan ultrasonography shows that the sclera is in fact usually thickened in active scleritis.

In elderly patients evidence of previous attacks should be sought. These present as patches of darkening due to translucency of the sclera, formerly called 'sclero-malacia' before ultrasound techniques were available. The anterior segment, particularly under the upper lid, should be examined. There may be confusion in elderly patients with benign hyaline degeneration in which regularly shaped rectangles of translucency appear adjacent to the insertions of the medial and lateral rectus muscles (*Fig.* 5.5).

Management: Scleritis in RA is evidence of widespread vasculitis and a poor prognosis for life. It is incurable, and when it occurs in an elderly rheumatoid patient will probably represent a recurrence of activity. Until recently initial attacks could be treated with oxyphenbutazone for a week, followed by systemic steroids if there was no response; oxyphenbutazone has now been withdrawn because of potentially harmful side-effects, and systemic steroids remain as the mainstay of management. The dose must vary according to the severity of the attack and the ability of the patient to withstand treatment. Generally 80–100 mg of prednisolone per day for a week, followed by slow reduction over a month may be recommended. In addition, topical steroids and mydriatics are indicated because of accompanying uveitis. In the absence of response or in the face of frequent recurrences, azathioprine (5 mg per kg body weight, and finally around 50 mg per day) may work wonders, at least for a few years.

There are rare instances of true scleral thinning requiring some form of surgical repair; most ophthalmologists see one case in a lifetime. Fascia lata, donor sclera or cornea and aortic tissue are among some of the materials recommended. The author has used a pedicle of adjacent healthy sclera to cover the gap and has closed over the pedicle area by approximating the edges of the healthy sclera with mattress suturing.

Summary: Scleritis is not a common disease and for it to start *de novo* in an elderly patient is extremely rare. In RA it points to the presence of widespread vasculitis and the prognosis is poor. Management revolves around steroids and other immunosuppressive agents.

UVEITIS AND OTHER DISORDERS

Inflammation of the iris, ciliary body or choroid in young adults and children may indicate the presence of a CTD, such as ankylosing spondylitis, Reiter's syndrome or juvenile RA. However, it is not a feature of adult RA, and it would be fruitless to search for a CTD in an elderly patient presenting with uveitis for the first time.

An astonishing array of ocular involvement in CTD has been recorded. With the exception of giant cell arteritis (*see* pp. 111, 129), none of these diseases has a high incidence in the elderly population. In systemic lupus erythematosus and progressive systemic sclerosis, unilateral proptosis, optic neuritis, branch arteriole or vein occlusion, non-specific keratopathy, upper lid and fornix shortening, and sectional atrophy of the dilator papillae and iris stroma have been reported.

LID ABNORMALITIES

'Entropion' means inturned, 'ectropion' means out-turned eyelid. Both contribute to or result from chronic conjunctivitis, and it may be impossible to tell which came first.

Entropion

This disorder can present in either upper or lower lid, but more commonly in the latter. 'Spastic' entropion accompanies an attack of conjunctivitis, and may resolve when the infection is controlled. It presents as an intermittent inturning of the lower eyelid, and can be demonstrated by getting the patient to close the eye tightly; she is then asked to open the eye, and it can be seen that the eyelid margin remains inturned.

Intermittent entropion may not require surgery. Topical antibiotics such as chloramphenicol, drops 0·5 per cent four times daily, and ointment night and morning over a week may cure the condition. In addition the eyelid margin may be taped down to the skin of the cheek, causing a deliberate ectropion, until the infection subsides.

Persistent entropion requires surgery. Various operations may be recommended according to the surgeon's experience and expertise. Most are successful, but repeat procedures are not uncommon.

Ectropion

The most common form in the elderly is senile ectropion, associated with atonicity of muscle and skin. Only the lower lid is affected. Trauma, e.g. burns and wounds, sometimes self-inflicted, though common in the young, are very uncommon in this age-group.

Unlike entropion, ectropion must be treated surgically if it is to be cured. However, it is necessary to consider whether the elderly patient is suffering as a result of the out-turned eyelid. In patients who do not have epiphora, the coexistence of dry eyes (*see above*) should be sought. If the ectropion eye is not watery, correction of the lid abnormality will not cure this form of 'conjunctivitis'. If the eye is watery, free drainage of tears through the nasolacrimal canaliculi into and through the tear sac must be established by a sac washout procedure. If these passages are blocked, again correction of the ectropion will not cure the watery eye. Nevertheless surgery may be recommended in all cases of ectropion to prevent the added insult of eye exposure.

As in the case of entropion there is a variety of operations each tailored to meet the patient's needs and the surgeon's experience. Repeat operations are rarely necessary.

Trichiasis

In-growing eyelashes should not be confused with entropion. The simplest management is epilation of the offending lashes, but these will recur in six weeks, and will be at their most irritating when they are tiny and almost invisible. In the elderly up to four lashes may be epilated repeatedly, usually by a nurse or relative accustomed to the procedure. Persistence of symptoms or extension of involvement of aberrant lashes requires a permanent solution. Diathermy to the lash roots is often successful, but in other patients the lash root follicles have to be transposed to another section of the eyelid away from the lid margin. The success of these operations depends on the speed with which the patient is referred to the ophthalmologist. If the trichiasis is long-standing and extensive, with more than half the lid margin excoriated and distorted, it is unlikely that a surgical cure will be obtained.

LACRIMAL (TEAR) DRAINAGE

Tears drain through the nasolacrimal canaliculi into the sac, and thence through its lower end into the nose. Epiphora may be the result of poor lid apposition to the tear film, as in ectropion or entropion, or because of blockage in the tear passages.

Canalicular Block

This can be determined only by scintigraphy. Forcible washing through of the tear passages can give a false impression of patency. In scintigraphy radio-active material is instilled into the lower fornix, and its progress through to the nose monitored by scanning. The point of blockage is readily determined, the solution to the problem is another matter. Reparative surgery to blocked canaliculi is rarely successful, and the physician would do well to consider the probable benefit to his patient before recommending surgery.

Sac Blockage

Acute dacryocystitis presents dramatically with the formation of an abscess in the lacrimal sac (*Fig.* 5.9). Immediate treatment in a toxic patient is with systemic antibiotics. Once the acute attack has subsided removal of the sac is normally recommended. The eye will remain watery.

Chronic dacryocystitis due to repeated low grade infection is one of the causes of chronic epiphora. Depending on the distress to the patient, surgery may be advised. Success is only some 50 per cent, and the operation of dacryocystorrhinostomy is taxing for the elderly patient. Many ophthalmologists will not undertake the procedure in patients over the age of 70.

Nasal Blockage

On occasion epiphora is due to enlarged or distorted nasal turbinates. This usually occurs in the young suffering from allergic rhinitis, but it should be considered in the elderly as the result of long-standing 'catarrh'. Cure may be effected by the removal of the excess or distorted nasal tissue.

LID CANCERS

Basal and squamous celled epitheliomas are common on the eyelids, comprising some 10–15 per cent of all cutaneous cancers. There is some controversy as to the highest peak incidence but it is generally agreed most occur between 50 and 70 years of age and that the disease is relatively uncommon in octogenarians. However, it should be borne in mind as a differential diagnosis in persistently recurrent lid 'cysts' in the elderly (*Plate III* 2) and as a possible contributor to lid distortion, either entropion or ectropion.

Management: Surgical excision is the accepted mode of treatment. There is no place for irradation of these tumours since deleterious involvement of the eye is virtually certain. On the other hand inner canthus spread to the lacrimal sac and ethmoid sinuses may warrant radiotherapy.

SUMMARY

Conjunctivitis is common in the elderly, and when persistent underlying causes such as the dry eye, lid malfunction, and abnormalities of nasolacrimal drainage should be considered. All of these are either completely remediable or at least eminently treatable.

FURTHER READING

Abdel-Khalen L. M. R., Williamson J. and Lee W. R. (1978) *Br. J. Ophthalmol.* **92,** 800.

Block J. H. J., Buchanan W. W., Woo N. J. and Burium J. J. (1965) *Medicine* (*Baltimore*) **44**, 187.

Damato B. E., Allan D., Murray S. B. and Lee W. R. (1984) *Br. J. Ophthalmol.* **68**, 674.

Van Rood J. J. (1984) *Ann. Rheum. Dis.* **43**, 665.

Watson P. G. and Hazleman B. L. (1976) *The Sclera and Systemic Disorders: Major Problems in Ophthalmology* Vol. 2. London, Saunders.

6. THE AGEING LENS
J. Dudgeon

The lens of the human eye is unique in a number of ways, containing the highest concentration of protein and glutathione of any tissue in the body. It is composed of one epithelial cell type only, contains a low water concentration relative to other tissues, and goes on increasing steadily in size throughout life as the old cells cannot be shed. Its thickness may increase from around 3·5 mm at birth to 5 mm in the eighties. The gradual increase in lens thickness is accompanied by increasing shallowness of the anterior chamber of the eye, and narrowing of the drainage angle, thus predisposing to the development of acute angle-closure glaucoma in the elderly.

The lens is transparent and biconvex in shape in adult life with the anterior surface less steeply curved than the posterior. It has been assumed since the time of Donders (1864), on theoretical grounds, that the lens flattened with age. The postulated progressive flattening of the anterior lens surface coupled with a hardening of the outer layer of the lens was invoked to explain the slow development of hypermetropia after middle age. Recent measurements, however, indicate an increase in the curvature of the anterior lens surface with age, rather than a decrease, and a progressive decrease in the posterior curvature.

Placed immediately behind the pupil with the posterior surface of the iris resting on it, the lens is surrounded by a capsule from the 13 mm embryonic stage onwards. The capsule is thicker anteriorly than posteriorly and increases in thickness with age, a factor which may have some bearing on the development and location of cataract. It doubles in thickness to 16μ by the age of 40. The capsule is composed of an inner homogeneous cuticular layer and an outer lamellar structure and is permeable to water, crystalloids, and to proteins of low molecular weight such as haemoglobin. The anterior capsule may show exfoliation of its outer lamellae in old age, forming thin sheet-like material visible in the pupil. This is to be distinguished from pseudo-exfoliation of the lens capsule in which there is deposition of greyish-white material on the anterior lens capsule, the iris, and the drainage angle of the anterior chamber, as in the latter condition there may be associated chronic glaucoma.

The permeability of the lens capsule decreases with age and has been shown to be the same in cataractous lenses and in normal lenses of age-matched controls, so that senile cataract is not due to an increase in capsular permeability, although it is well known that traumatic tears in the capsule readily cause opacification of the lens. The elastic strength of the capsule decreases with age, a factor which may play a part in the development of presbyopia. The lens which weighs about 65 mg at birth has doubled its weight by the end of the first year of life, and by the 9th decade it has doubled its weight once more.

The lens needs metabolic energy in the form of energy-rich compounds for the maintenance of its transparency. These compounds, e.g. ATP, ADP, are provided by carbohydrate metabolism which takes the form of anaerobic glycolysis in the lens fibres which have lost their mitochondria. Oxidative phosphorylation, which is confined to the single layer of epithelial cells at the front of the lens, also contributes significantly to lens metabolism. The metabolic activity of the lens shows a progressive decrease with age. The whole of glycolytic enzyme activity lessens, and the hexose monophosphate pathway in particular is profoundly diminished.

Deficiency of essential amino acids is known to lead to the production of cataract, but only during the period of deficiency, since as soon as a normal diet is restored clear lens fibres are laid down again. The tripeptide glutathione, present in high concentration in the lens, is of great importance for various biochemical functions such as the elimination of peroxides or radicals occurring as the result of physical influences. An adequate supply of glutathione is dependent on an adequate amino acid supply. The processes leading to lens opacities mostly involve a decrease in glutathione content even before changes in transparency occur.

During the ageing process a decrease in the energy supply in the lens occurs, due to the fact that some enzymes catalysing energy-providing reactions are subjected to post-translational changes which cause a slowing down of the reaction course. Two enzymes in particular are subject to such age-related changes:
1. Hexokinase, which catalyses phosphorylation of glucose to glucose-6-phosphate.
2. Phosphofructokinase, which catalyses phosphorylation of fructose-6-phosphate to fructose, 1,6-diphosphate.

Other enzymes showing lowered activity are aldolase, carbonic anhydrase, and various dehydrogenases. Chemical changes in the lens with age involve a decrease in potassium and phosphates, and in the sulphur-containing cysteine and glutathione. The levels of ascorbic acid and water also fall, while sodium and calcium levels rise, as do the levels of free and total cholesterol.

LENS PROTEINS

Thirty-five per cent of the lens is composed of organic matter which is mainly structural proteins (α, β, γ, crystallins and the insoluble protein fraction). The protein concentration in the lens is higher than it is in any other tissue, the concentration in the nucleus being greater than that in the cortex. The total protein content increases with age. The most important change in this respect is an increase in the insoluble (albuminoid) proteins from a level of 6–7 per cent of the total protein in youth to 67 per cent in old age. The water-soluble crystallins show a concomitant decrease, as the synthesis of soluble protein decreases as well as the activity of amino acids, RNA, and protein- incorporation systems.

It has been postulated that the high concentration of protein in the lens may have a barrier effect against the influx of water and ions towards the inner regions of the lens. If this is so, then a breakdown of this barrier may lead to gradual lens hydration—a factor in the process of lens opacification and the formation of certain types of cataract. One possible reason for such a barrier breakdown might be the slow qualitative age-related change in lens cystallins due to their enzymatic and random hydrolytic breakdown. Loss of crystallins due to 'leak out' has also been reported.

The vertebrate lens probably contains the body's longest lived proteins. The lens is therefore a suitable organ for studying the effect of ageing on proteins *in vivo*. Lens metabolism in general is very slow compared to other mammalian tissues. There is practically no protein turnover in the nucleus of the lens which has little or no protease activity. Because of their long lifespan the lens proteins may be highly vulnerable to damage. Accumulation of faulty protein is a universal phenomenon of ageing, and a high incidence in the ageing lens of defective proteins, formed by postsynthetic changes, has been observed.

The concentration of dry mass, which is almost exclusively protein, determines the refractive index and the refractive properties of the lens. In a normal lens, protein distribution is even within each layer; a smooth gradient from one layer to another occurs so that apart from the immediate subcapsular layer there is a slight but progressive increase in refractive index, especially in the nucleus. Uneven distribution of protein gives rise to 'jumps' in refractive index. Such fluctuations (optical anisotropy) provide for an increase in light scattering. High molecular weight aggregates, which are dense, increase with ageing on a weight/volume basis leading to an increase in refractive index difference between the aggregates and their surroundings.

Optical anisotropy fluctuations increasingly contribute more scattered light with ageing due to a decrease in size and misalignment of the birefringent cytoskeletal bodies. An increased component of light scattering with age is thus due to an increase in the total birefringence.

Density fluctuations, however, are more important in producing light scattering than are fluctuations in optical anisotropy. Density fluctuations are caused by a combined aggregation-syneresis process. During this process protein molecules aggregate by intermolecular crosslinking, by primary valence bonds such as disulphide bridges, by ionic bridges, by hydrophobic interactions, and by hydrogen bonding.

Increased light scattering with age is one of the factors producing reduced illuminance in older eyes. Other factors are senile miosis and the presence of a yellow pigment in the lens which absorbs short wavelengths. The retina of the aged eye receives less light in general and less blue-violet radiation in particular than the youthful retina. It has been estimated that the retina of the average 60-year-old receives about one-third of the light received by the retina of the average 20-year-old. It is very important, therefore, to ensure that the elderly use a source of bright illumination when reading, etc., and to remember to position the lighting close to the object to be illuminated because of the rapid fall off in light intensity the further away the light (inverse square law).

It is now generally agreed that chronic exposure to ultraviolet radiation (300–400 nm) over an individual's lifetime leads to the generation and increased accumulation of various fluorescent chromophores in the lens which are to some extent responsible for the increased yellow colour of the lens nucleus. Such an accumulation of pigment in the lens nucleus produces a reduction in light transmission, as it acts as a coloured filter in front of the eye.

There are no chromophores in the young lens capable of absorbing radiation longer than 295 nm, apart from a minute amount of cytochromes in the lens epithelial cells. The potential for absorbing u.v. radiation longer than 295 nm resides mainly in the tryptophan residues present in the lens proteins plus the relatively small amount of free tryptophan in the lens. Ultraviolet radiation is a significant factor in the generation of the fluorescent compounds, and in protein cross-linking associated with lens ageing and cataractogenesis in mouse, rat, rabbit, and primate lenses. Human u.v. radiation cataracts have been described.

The human lens is constantly exposed to ambient u.v. radiation throughout life as the cornea and aqueous transmit almost all u.v. radiation longer than 300 nm, although there is a progressive decrease in the percentage transmitted as the individual ages. At sea level u.v. radiation varies from 1–5 mw/cm² depending on geographic location and season. The sun is the main source of such radiation. The spectral output of fluorescent lamps in common use is relatively low between 295 and 400 nm, and therefore does not constitute a problem except for those who are taking photosensitising drugs.

As the lens ages it seems that there is an increase in the formation of fluorescent chromophores due to u.v. radiation. In theory an ultraviolet-induced free radical mechanism is involved with tryptophan acting as the absorbing chromophore. The high concentration of glutathione in the cortex acts to prevent the free radical-induced photochemical generation of these fluorescent chromophores. The lens nucleus has a much lower concentration of glutathione, and therefore a less effective protective mechanism, so that photochemically-induced pigments are generated, leading to an age-related increase in yellow-brown coloration of the nucleus as it ages.

Perhaps the decrease in the amount of light reaching the retina in the elderly eye contributes to the fact that many older individuals have an impaired ability to detect larger objects, despite adequate levels of acuity as conventionally measured, and a need for much greater contrast to detect low spatial frequencies. Whatever the mechanism responsible for this phenomenon, clear print with a sharp contrast between the letters and the page on which they lie is needed by the elderly. Black on white or white on black are therefore to be preferred, and coloured forms of notepaper, while fashionable, are nonetheless best avoided.

CHANGES IN ACCOMMODATION

An invariable change with increasing age is a decline in the amplitude of accommodation, which is the ability of the eye to increase its power to converge light. This decrease in accommodation (presbyopia) is thought to be multifactorial in aetiology but lens changes play an important role. There is a reduction in the volume of the nucleus relative to the entire lens, since the width of the nucleus remains constant with age while the width of the cortex increases. The nucleus plays an active role during accommodation in changing the shape of the lens, becoming markedly thickened, thus producing an increase in the anterior lens curvature and an increase in the focusing power of the eye. With age its function is relatively reduced because the nucleus is relatively smaller.

In addition there is an age-related reduction in capsular elasticity, doubtless contributing significantly to loss of accommodation, and possibly associated with loss of microlamellae from this thickest basement membrane in the body. There is considerable variation in the age of onset of presbyopia, depending on factors such as the basic refractive state of the eye, the amount of close work normally undertaken, etc. As the near point for easily sustained clear vision recedes, spectacles become necessary, usually as the mid to late forties in Western countries. There is a suggestion of an association between age onset of presbyopia and life expectancy, and a statistical correlation was demonstrated by Weale (1982) on the basis of the published figures.

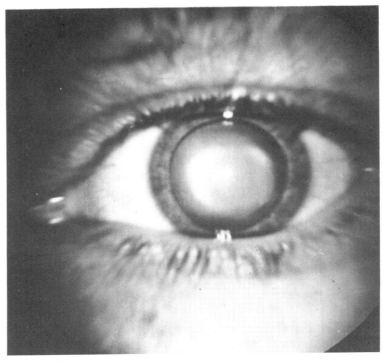

Fig. 6.1. Nuclear sclerosis.

between age of onset of presbyopia and ambient temperature—the higher the temperature, the earlier the onset of presbyopia.

The decrease in accommodative power with age gradually increases, so that one of the commonest causes of visual handicap among the elderly is a need for new reading glasses. Surveys show this to be the case in as many as 40 per cent of those in geriatric institutions, a population who are known not to be given to complaining about reduced vision. Routine testing of these individuals and the prescription of accurate spectacles would therefore seem to be a useful exercise.

LENS OPACITIES

Different forms of lens opacities are found with ageing and may involve predominantly the nucleus, the cortex, or the posterior subcapsular zone, or may occur in mixed forms. To label all of these as 'senile cataract' is incorrect and supports the idea that ageing alone is responsible for the opacification, whereas the pathogenesis of senile cataract is multifactorial. Nuclear opacity (*Fig.* 6.1) is associated with

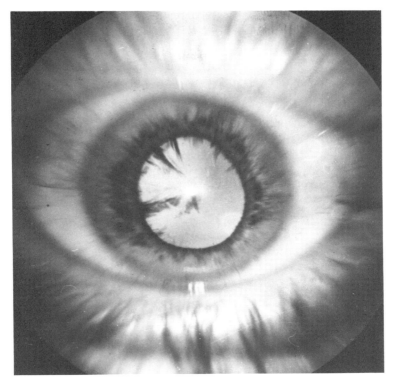

Fig. 6.2. Peripheral cortical opacities.

sclerosis with an increase in refractive index which produces a myopic change in the eye. The patient may find as a consequence that she can read unaided again, while the distance vision may improve with a minus spectacle correction. Posterior subcapsular opacities (*Plate IV*) have an effect on vision out of proportion to their density by virtue of their position, and may necessitate early lens extraction. Peripheral cortical opacities (*Fig.* 6.2) may contribute to dazzling in bright light, and to multiple image formation, but will not reduce visual acuity until they encroach on the visual axis.

It is not possible to clear senile lens opacities but the question remains as to whether or not one might avoid, delay, or stop the process leading to opacification. Numerous preparations are on offer, especially on the Continent of Europe, but there is no evidence that any of these commercial products are effective. Substances intended to inhibit the enzyme aldose reductase are under investigation for their clinical use in inhibiting cataract formation. The reasoning behind their use is that true diabetic cataract is due to the formation of the sugar alcohol sorbitol. This polyol is formed from glucose by aldose reductase and accumulates in the lens, disturbing its osmotic equilibrium, and causing an influx of water, intumescence, and opacification of the lens. The mechanism is also active in the formation of polyols from galactose, xylose, or arabinose. True diabetic cataract, however, is rare and occurs over a period of five to seven days, a situation quite unlike that occurring in typical senile cataract.

It is interesting that in established diabetes there is an abnormally rapid rate of growth of the lens, almost entirely due to an increase in width of the cortex, so that the dimensions of the lens of the diabetic come to resemble those of a normal subject sixteen years older. Perhaps the excessive size of the diabetic lens is causally linked to the development of cataract in diabetics, which occurs about ten years earlier than in normal subjects.

Acetylsalicylic acid has been reported as causing a delay in cataract formation, but such reports await further confirmation. It is postulated that a possible mode of action of acetylsalicyclic acid may be by a reduction in plasma levels of bound tryptophan, which it lowers by as much as 50 per cent. Increased tryptophan levels have been reported in the plasma of cataract patients.

Processes leading to lens opacities mostly involve a decrease in glutathione content even before changes in transparency occur. It is known that glycine, glutamic acid, and cysteine all lead to an increase in glutathione concentration *in vitro,* but there is no evidence of any effect in reducing lens opacities in patients by their use. It is interesting, however, that glutathione synthesis is dependent on an adequate amino acid supply, and that there is evidence from epidemiological studies that low total protein consumption is a risk factor that may account for as much as 40 per cent of the excess prevalence of cataract in areas such as the Punjab.

PSEUDOEXFOLIATION OF THE LENS CAPSULE

This condition is characterized by the deposition of an abnormal basement membrane material, with amyloid-like characteristics, on the anterior lens capsule. The material is also deposited on the iris, in the drainage angle of the anterior chamber, and indeed even in extra-ocular sites. It is recognized clinically as flecks of greyish, fluffy material in the pupillary aperture (*Fig.* 6.3).

There is a clear increase of this condition with increasing age so that about 7 per cent of the over-seventies are affected. The condition occurs all over the world and among all races, but an hereditary factor is probably of some significance as evidenced by increased prevalence among certain population groups. There is a definite association with

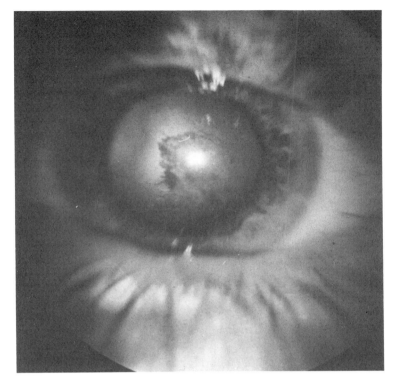

Fig. 6.3. Pseudoexfoliation.

open-angle glaucoma with as many as 22 per cent of affected individuals showing evidence of this disease, which is often more severe and more difficult to control than classical primary open-angle glaucoma.

REFERENCES

Weale R. A. (1982) *A Biography of the Eye.* London, H. K. Lewis.

FURTHER READING

Bloemendal H. (ed.) (1981) *Molecular and Cellular Biology of the Eye Lens.* New York, Wiley.

Duncan G. (ed.) (1981) *Mechanisms of Cataract Formation in the Human Lens.* London, Academic Press.

Elliott K. and Fitzsimmons D. W. (eds) (1973) *The Human Lens—in relation to Cataract.* Ciba Foundation Symposium **19** (new series). Amsterdam, Elsevier, North-Holland.

Regnault F., Hockwin O., and Courtois Y. (eds) (1980) *Ageing of the Lens.* Amsterdam, Elsevier, North-Holland.

7. CATARACT
A. L. Crombie

Different mechanisms appear to trigger off loss of transparency of the lens in different types of cataract (*see* Chapters 2 *and* 6). Cortical senile cataract (*see below*) is characterized by an early monovalent cation shift, and nuclear cataract by the insolubilization and colouration of structural proteins. Clayton et al. (1982) examined some risk factors associated with cataract and found that age, diabetes and the use of diuretics were associated with it, and an association between hypertension and cataract has now emerged from three independent studies. There is much interest in sugar-induced cataracts, not only because of those which occur, e.g. in galactosaemia, but because it is believed that the same mechanisms may be partly implicated in the development of senile and pre-senile cataracts in patients who are not diabetic.

Cataracts may be classified in many ways but in senile cataract classification by the anatomical site seems to correlate more clearly with symptoms than any other. There are thus four main groups—cortical, nuclear, capsular (anterior or posterior), and sub-capsular (anterior or posterior). In relation to the development of visual symptoms each can be subdivided into a further two groups, stationary or progressive.

COMMON SYMPTOMS

Many old people who suffer from cataracts do not describe any symptoms, but are referred to an ophthalmologist because the cataract has been found incidentally, either by another medical practitioner or by an optician. It is surprising how many older patients expect to have poor vision, and do not seek help until visual symptoms are very marked. The most common symptom of cataract is failing vision, which will be greatest in diffuse or posterior polar cataract, and least in cataracts involving the periphery of the lens. In nuclear cataracts the centre of the lens often becomes myopic; the patient has no problems with reading vision but has significant problems in the distance. When the opacities are in the visual axis, the patient often sees better in dim illumination because the dilated pupil allows her to see through the clearer periphery. Another common symptom is photophobia, which is related to the

70

scattering of light by the opacities in the lens somewhat akin to the sun shining on a dirty car windscreen. Patients may also complain of blank spots (positive scotomata) in the visual field. Their position remains fixed when the eye is moved and they are most noticeable against an evenly bright background. They differ from vitreous opacities in their lack of movement when the eye moves. Some patients complain of uniocular polyopia, often seeing two or three images with one eye, due to the refraction from scattered lens opacities. In addition cataracts may also give rise to halos around lights which can, at times, be mistaken for those occurring in acute angle-closure glaucoma. A discerning patient may also complain of changes in colour values, since under normal circumstances the lens absorbs more of the blue end of the spectrum than the red, and as the lens becomes cataractous all the blue shades are absorbed, so that orange colours predominate.

DIAGNOSIS

The diagnosis of cataract can be made objectively. The principal sign is a whitish opacity within the pupillary area. The colour of the opacity may vary from white to grey, to a very light grey sheen, or may be difficult to discern because it is dark and does not cause any light scattering within the pupil. Such dark cataracts, however, are immediately visible in the beam of a slit lamp or an ophthalmoscope. When the pupil is dilated, transillumination shows up lens opacities very well as black silhouettes against the background red reflex of the fundus. Their location either at the periphery or at the centre is easily diagnosed with a simple ophthalmoscope, whilst their position in the antero-posterior diameter is more easily determined on a slit lamp examination.

EVALUATION OF VISUAL FUNCTION

Visual failure is the main reason for cataract evaluation and surgery. It is important to try and ascertain whether a good visual result may be expected following surgery. Details of the techniques involved are provided in Chapter 4.

The use of ultrasonography has made the evaluation of an eye with a dense cataract more satisfactory in terms of possible other pathologies, since vitreous haemorrhage, intra-ocular tumours and retinal detachments can be correctly diagnosed non-invasively (McLeod et al., 1977).

There have been many electro-physiological studies carried out to determine the integrity of macular function. Unfortunately, electro-retinography (ERG) provides only a mass response. It has not yet been possible to use this technique except to show that the retina as a whole is functional (Ponte et al., 1981). The visual evoked potential (VEP;

sometimes called 'visual evoked responses' (VER)) is the average electrical response from the visual cortex to repeated light stimulation. Because the macular area of the retina is more heavily represented in the visual cortex than the periphery, the electrical response recorded can be related fairly closely to visual acuity. Macular degeneration, optic atrophy or amblyopia will produce an abnormal VEP, whereas a cataract alone will give a normal reading (Thompson and Harding, 1977).

Reduced Visual Function

The main indication for cataract extraction is reduced visual acuity because of cataract. When the degree of visual impairment is severe the indication for surgery is usually clear-cut. For lesser degrees of visual impairment a qualitative decision has to be reached between the surgeon and the patient as to whether the ratio of benefit to risk is favourable.

Other indications for cataract removal are 'medical'. They include swelling of the lens causing a shallow anterior chamber with resultant angle-closure glaucoma and leakage of lens matter from a hypermature lens causing uveitis (*see* Chapter 8).

CATARACT SURGERY

Pre-operative Assessment

An elderly patient admitted for cataract extraction needs to be assessed in two main ways: in relation to the eye itself (many of the ocular investigations will have been carried out in the out-patient department as detailed previously) and in relation to her general medical condition.

Approximately 60 per cent of elderly cataract extraction patients have a medical problem, the main ones being hypertension, cardiovascular disease, diabetes, chronic lung disease and rheumatoid arthritis (Gilvarry and Eustace, 1982). Haemoglobin, serum urea and potassium, urinalysis, fasting blood glucose, chest X-ray and ECG should be carried out on all patients prior to surgery, particularly if general anaesthesia is to be embarked upon; in the author's opinion it is as important that the patient is as fully worked up for local as for general anaesthesia. Once this has been done the eyelashes of the eye to be operated upon are cut, and routine local topical antibiotic therapy is instituted for 12 hours before surgery.

Anaesthesia

There are a number of basic requirements for ophthalmic anaesthesia. These include complete akinesia of the globe and lids, complete anaesthesia of the globe and adnexae, control of intra-ocular pressure and systemic blood pressure, relaxation of the patient, smooth induction and emergence from the anaesthetic state, and adequate postoperative analgesia. The decision has to be made as to whether the cataract should be removed under local or general anaesthesia. In recent times the only real contra-indication to general anaesthesia has been severe pulmonary disease. However, some patients opt for local anaesthesia, as do their families; if so, proper pre-operative sedation is necessary to ensure relaxation during the preparation for the introduction of local anaesthetic agents. The author uses 10 mg diazepam given some hours before; this not only produces relaxation but postoperative amnesia to a mild degree. Modern cataract surgery usually utilizes an operating microscope. It is often very difficult for an elderly person to lie completely still for up to thirty minutes. General anaesthesia is therefore becoming the rule in the United Kingdom. Control of the respiratory and cardiovascular systems is also easier during general anaesthesia

If local anaesthesia has been decided upon, surface anaesthesia should be induced by amethocaine 1 per cent or tetracaine 0·5 per cent. Akinesia is induced by blocking the branches of the facial nerve supplying the orbicularis muscle and the associated facial muscles; this can be effected by a series of injections in the lateral side of the orbit or just anterior to the temporomandibular joint. Akinesia of the extra-ocular muscles and anaesthesia of the conjunctiva, cornea and iris is effected by blocking the ciliary nerves, using a retrobulbar block in which the anaesthetic agent is injected within the muscle cone. This injection will also slow down optic nerve conduction and make the patient less visually aware of surgery.

Many massage the eye and surrounding tissues for approximately five minutes, following the regional and retrobulbar blocks, to ensure that the local anaesthetic has thoroughly permeated the tissues; some add hyaluronidase to the local injection to ensure that this happens as quickly as possible. A soft eye is a prerequisite for cataract surgery particularly when intra-ocular lenses are to be inserted. Massage by hand or by the use of a Harman bag may be helpful in this respect.

If general anaesthesia is to be used, the patient's drug therapy should be evaluated by the anaesthetist prior to surgery. He must ensure that the dosage of the drugs required is correct, and also preclude possible interactions between anaesthetic agents and the patient's drug regimen.

Pre-operative medication usually consists of atropine and a tranquil-lizer (e.g. diazepam). Anaesthesia is induced by intravenous sodium pentothal and succinylcholine. The patient may be maintained on nitrous oxide or halothane; the latter is usually preferred, since it provides rapid and easy emergence from anaesthesia and seems adequate with oxygen. It can, however, sensitize the heart to catechol-amines and repeated use of halothane may produce liver damage in those thought to have an allergy to it (Jacoby, 1976). The patient is hyperventilated to wash out carbon dioxide and decrease blood volume within the eye, thus causing the vitreous to shrink, and producing a soft eye. It is important that the patient emerges from general anaesthesia following cataract surgery as smoothly as possible. In particular coughing and vomiting should be avoided, since this raises the intra-ocular pressure and may rupture incisions or cause intra-ocular haemorrhage by raising the central venous pressure.

The incidence of complications following cataract surgery seems to be the same whether local anaesthesia or general anaesthesia is used, but it is worth remembering that one study has suggested that the death rate of patients undergoing eye surgery appears to be twice that of the general population matched for age (Breslin, 1973).

Surgery

After anaesthesia has been induced, by whatever method, the eye is opened by a corneo-scleral or corneal incision. There are then two methods open to the surgeon of removing a cataract:

1. The *intracapsular technique* by which the lens is removed *in toto* from the eye; and

2. The *extracapsular technique* whereby the anterior capsule, the nucleus and the cortex of the lens are removed, leaving the posterior capsule attached to form a barrier between the vitreous and the anterior segment of the eye.

Intracapsular extraction is a simpler technique and almost always results in complete removal of the lens but, on the other hand, the wound has to be slightly larger, there is a fair chance of corneal endothelial damage because of instrumentation or bending of the cornea during removal of the lens, and postoperative pupil block by the vitreous face may occur.

Extracapsular cataract surgery involves a smaller incision and a diminution in postoperative astigmatism, whilst the division between the vitreous and the anterior chamber is maintained and a secure base remains on which to support an intra-ocular lens (Rich, 1982). However, extracapsular surgery is more difficult than intracapsular, and a well-dilated pupil and deep anterior chamber must be maintained throughout the operation. In extracapsular surgery there may also be corneal endothelial damage either by instrumentation or fluid irrigation and late opacification of the posterior capsule causes further visual failure. There is no doubt that the extracapsular method is rapidly gaining favour, particularly because of the introduction of intra-ocular lens implantation, which is thought to be safer when the extracapsular method is used. The incidence of postoperative retinal detachment and cystoid macular oedema is also supposed to be less than with the intracapsular method (Rich, 1982).

Either method allows the removal of opaque lens matter obstructing the visual axis to allow clear passage of light to the retina. This is achieved in well over 90 per cent of cases using either method. In the intracapsular method the lens is removed using a cryo-extractor which causes an ice ball to form between the small frozen tip and the lens itself. This ensures a firm grip and reduces rupture of the capsule; it is the method of choice rather than grasping the lens with capsule forceps.

In the extracapsular method the anterior capsule is cut open by an irrigating cystotome and the nucleus of the lens manoeuvred into the anterior chamber and removed by mechanical means. The cortex of the lens is removed by gentle suction. Some surgeons, having cleaned the posterior capsule, perforate it in the area of the visual axis to reduce the possibility of interference with the light path to the macula. Damage to the corneal endothelium can be minimized if air or sodium hyaluronate is used in the anterior chamber to maintain its depth during these manoeuvres. Sodium hyaluronate may occasionally lead to a slightly raised postoperative intra-ocular pressure, but this is easily dealt with by systemic acetazolamide therapy for 24 hours. Intracapsular cataract removal can be facilitated by the use of alpha-chymotrypsin, which dissolves the zonular fibres holding the lens in place, and allows smoother removal of the lens.

Intra-ocular lens implantation has become very popular because of good postoperative visual results compared to other methods of correcting aphakic vision. There are three main groups of intra-ocular lenses:
1. *Those which lie in the anterior chamber* supported by 'feet' in the anterior chamber angle and which can be used in either intracapsular or extracapsular extractions,
2. *Iris-fixed lenses* where the lens is clipped to the iris and usually lies in the anterior chamber, and
3. *Posterior chamber lenses* (which are almost exclusively used in the extracapsular method) where the lens is supported by feet which extend into the recesses of the remaining capsule at its periphery.

At the present time approximately 30 per cent of implanted lenses are of the anterior chamber type, and 70 per cent of the posterior chamber type. Very few iris-supported lenses are now used, because of problems with movement of the lens, iris atrophy from mechanical trauma, and corneal endothelial cell damage (Galin et al., 1982). In both types of surgery monofilament continuous or interrupted sutures are used to close the corneal wound and are buried so that they cause no irritation and need not be removed.

Following surgery a topical antibiotic is instilled and a subconjunctival injection of antibiotic given. After this the eye is firmly padded and the patient remains in bed for 18–24 hours.

Complications of Cataract Surgery

The catalogue of complications following cataract surgery is long, but it must be remembered that the vast majority of cataract extractions are successful and that restoration of a reasonable degree of vision occurs in over 90 per cent. Complications can be divided into two main groups, those occurring during the operation and those occurring in the postoperative period.

The first serious complication which can occur during operation is the extremely rare expulsive haemorrhage. Once the eye has been opened and the tissue pressure reduced to nil, a massive infilling of the choroidal vessels occurs with haemorrhage beneath the retina. In the past this has usually been untreatable but, with rapid closure of the eye and evacuation of the blood, some degree of success in restoration of vision has been claimed. In the author's opinion expulsive haemorrhage still causes almost total visual loss.

A much more common complication occurring during surgery is vitreous loss. This occurs in between one and seven per cent of cases, almost exclusively in those who have an intracapsular cataract extraction. The anterior vitreous face may be ruptured during extraction of the lens or in manipulation of the iris. This is an indication for an anterior vitrectomy, i.e. the removal of the vitreous from the anterior chamber, so that none remains to cause wound leaks, corneal endothelial cell dysfunction, a peaked pupil or uveitis. The advent of vitreous surgery means that vitreous loss is no longer the catastrophe that it used to be, although it is still a complication to be avoided if at all possible. The use of general anaesthesia during which PCO_2 is reduced causes the eye to be soft and decreases the risk of vitreous loss. In cases in which the eye is myopic, and as a result the vitreous is degenerate, there is a higher than average incidence of vitreous loss even in the best hands.

One of the most feared complications of cataract surgery is bacterial endophthalmitis. The infection usually occurs while the eye is open and manifests itself within the first 24 hours by the appearance of oedema of the lids, a marked degree of conjunctival injection, pain, and the appearance of pus in the eye. Immediate measures have to be taken in the form of vigorous antibacterial therapy, the institution of systemic steroid treatment, and posterior vitrectomy in which all the infected vitreous is removed (Eichenbaum et al., 1978). The use of intravitreal antibiotic therapy (Davidson, 1984) has proved useful in preserving a degree of vision, but bacterial endophthalmitis is still a very serious complication, though occurring in only one in a thousand cases.

In the early postoperative period choroidal detachment, often associated with a flat anterior chamber, is usually the consequence of a corneal wound leak. Conservative treatment includes firm padding of the eye in the hope of sealing the wound and the reduction of intra-ocular pressure with acetazolamide. Whilst choroidal detachment usually in itself causes no harm, the flattening of the anterior chamber may cause peripheral anterior synechiae to form. These in turn may cause a secondary aphakic glaucoma, particularly if the anterior chamber has remained flat for more than 48 hours and two-thirds of the circumference of the angle is involved. Another cause of flat anterior chamber is aphakic pupillary block, in which the intra-ocular pressure rises markedly because the vitreous face has moved forwards and becomes adherent to the iris. The vitreous then plugs the pupillary opening as well as the iridectomy openings. In this type of flat anterior chamber the intra-ocular pressure is usually markedly raised, whereas in the flat anterior chamber due to a corneal wound leak the pressure is low. Conservative treatment consists of dilating the pupil as widely as possible and the use of systemic acetazolamide in the first instance. If the intra-ocular pressure is not normalized within the first 24 hours, vitrectomy is indicated to remove the vitreous plug from the pupillary area and thus normalize the flow of aqueous humour.

Occasionally, if the corneal incision is not totally sealed there may be iris prolapse, in which a small piece of iris becomes plugged in the incision. This usually causes a peaked pupil and often a low-grade uveitis which may impair the return of reasonable vision. If iris prolapse occurs early, surgical repair is necessary, but if it is a late phenomenon it can be more difficult to repair surgically, but the degree of uveitis may be minimal.

Corneal oedema following cataract surgery often occurs because of irritation of the anterior chamber and mechanical trauma to the cells of the corneal endothelium. This usually lasts a few days and settles spontaneously but if it persists it may be due to vitreous touching the posterior surface of the cornea and causing endothelial cell dysfunction. In such cases topical hyperosmotic therapy can be used, but occasionally anterior vitrectomy may be needed to clear the vitreous and allow the corneal endothelium to return to normal function.

A rare complication nowadays following cataract surgery is the ingrowth of epithelial cells from the surface of the eye into the anterior chamber through a small corneal wound dehiscence. With the advent of better suturing material and microscopical aids, this complication is now rare but can still occur. When it does, removal of the epithelial cells from within the anterior chamber is necessary if some degree of reasonable vision is to ensue. This may be done by using cryotherapy to the cornea to kill the cells lining its posterior surface.

A very common complication affecting the macular area, cystoid macular oedema, occurs in approximately 90 per cent of cases but resolves spontaneously in most. It is sometimes associated with vitreous loss and intra-ocular lens implantation, as well as certain topical drugs such as adrenaline. It usually occurs some 6–8 weeks after cataract extraction, and is often asymptomatic, but some patients complain of impaired visual acuity following reasonable acuity initially. Fluorescein angiography can delineate the degree of oedema, but there is no specific treatment (Rosen, 1975). Its pathogenesis may in part be related to traction on the macula by the vitreous or hypotony at the time of operation, but a common finding is a low-grade uveitis characterized by flare (protein) in the anterior chamber and a cellular reaction in the posterior vitreous. Most cases resolve spontaneously, but a small percentage go on to develop macular degeneration.

Postoperative retinal detachment occurs in 1–2 per cent of cases, mostly within the first two years and particularly within the first six months. Patients who have myopia or have had a retinal detachment in the fellow eye or have retinal lattice degeneration are at a higher risk. Vitreous loss is an important factor in aphakic detachment, though with the advent of vitrectomy this complication may be reduced in the future. The pathogenesis of this type of retinal detachment seems to be a forward shift of the vitreous causing a series of small retinal breaks at the posterior border of its base. It may also be due to zonular lens fibres mechanically disturbing the peripheral retina especially after intra-capsular extraction. Aphakic retinal detachments occur most often in the superior half of the retina, the majority of holes being in the upper temporal quadrant closely followed by the upper nasal (Jaffe, 1981). Pre-operative cryotherapy in patients with myopia and peripheral retinal degenerations may help to decrease the incidence of postoperative retinal detachment. As with all retinal detachments, it is important that the condition be diagnosed as soon as possible. Cryotherapy and scleral implant should be embarked upon before the macula is detached, since once this happens the chances of reasonable central vision being restored are greatly lessened.

In extracapsular extraction approximately 10 per cent of patients develop secondary membranes ('after cataract'). The posterior capsule thickens and surgery is needed to restore an intact light path.

The presence of an implanted lens predisposes to a greater degree of uveitis. There is increasing evidence of corneal endothelial dysfunction some years after, possibly because of loss of cells at the time of operation. This is a quite different type of corneal oedema from that in the immediate postoperative period, which is usually due to mechanical trauma to the corneal endothelium, and it can only be treated by corneal transplantation (Cheng, 1983). There is also an increased incidence of secondary glaucoma either due to inflammatory cells blocking the outflow channels in the irido-corneal angle or as a direct result of mechanical trauma to the angle caused by the 'feet' of the anterior chamber intra-ocular lenses.

Iris supported lenses have an increased incidence of iris atrophy and pigment deposition on the cornea due to mechanical trauma. The presence of an intra-ocular lens can, on occasion, make visualization of the retina difficult, particularly when the peripheral retina needs to be seen in relation to a postoperative retinal detachment.

Despite all these complications, uncomplicated cataract extraction is the rule. It is quite in order to predict good visual results in the majority, once a good pre-operative work-up has excluded other ocular disease.

REHABILITATION

The length of stay in hospital because of cataract extraction has been markedly reduced in recent years, and now ranges from one to four days. Within 24 hours of surgery, the patient should be sitting up and moving normally to minimize chest complications and the risks of pulmonary emboli. Any pain or discomfort should have subsided within the first 24 hours. Topical treatment to dilate the pupil is usually necessary except where a constricted pupil is needed to support an iris clip lens. Topical antibiotic treatment is needed to minimize any postoperative infection, whilst topical steroid treatment is necessary for a period of some weeks since a low grade traumatic uveitis is always present. If the patient has had an intra-ocular lens implantation reasonable vision should be present within 48 hours and should gradually improve. Otherwise temporary aphakic glasses can be prescribed, which may at least allow the patient to become reorientated in her surroundings to a limited extent, or a contact lens will give reasonable vision within a very short time of operation. Most patients having cataract surgery are elderly, and may well be disorientated in hospital and take longer than a younger patient to return to 'normal' even within their own home environment. Extra help is necessary from relatives or voluntary or statutory agencies. Limited physical activity is recommended for at least a period of two weeks to allow reasonable wound healing and to minimize the incidence of early postoperative complications.

After intra-ocular lens implantation reading glasses should be prescribed some six to eight weeks after surgery. If the patient's unoperated eye has reasonable vision, an intra-ocular lens may restore binocularity with a good field of vision, but some patients may complain of blurring of vision due to a slight shift in the position of the intra-ocular lens causing changes in refraction. Pseudophakic patients may complain of photophobia, possibly due to changes in absorption of light by the intra-ocular as compared to the normal lens.

There are two main ways of restoring vision to patients who have had a lens extraction without intra-ocular lens implantation. The first involves the prescription of aphakic glasses usually between 6 and 8 weeks postoperatively, when the final shape of the cornea is known. Aphakic spectacles are hypermetropic and are of high power. The intrinsic properties of these lenses are such that they magnify images of approximately 30 per cent and limit the field of vision because of the optical properties of the periphery of the lens. The result is that the patient has difficulty in judging distances because of the change in image size, and there is a smaller field of vision than normal. Approximately 95 per cent of patients adapt to aphakic spectacles, but 5 per cent never do and complain bitterly of the difficulties in judging distance and the degree of peripheral distortion and loss of field which can, at times, even induce vomiting. It is therefore very important to fit the spectacles correctly. Modern aspheric lenses reduce the problem of peripheral distortion to a large extent.

The second method of restoring vision is the use of contact lenses. Two main types of lenses are used, hard micro lenses and the somewhat larger soft lenses. Either causes image magnification of between 5 and 7 per cent, which does not cause a problem in judging distance. Soft contact lenses cannot correct higher degrees of astigmatism and can cause peripheral corneal vascularization and allergic conjunctivitis. They are, however, easier to manipulate for an older person, and some of the newer types can be left for up to three months at a time. In most cases spectacles also need to be prescribed for reading. Hard lenses, on the other hand, are much more difficult to manipulate but can correct higher degrees of astigmatism and are not so fragile. Adaptation to hard lenses is more difficult than to soft, but after cataract surgery there may be a degree of corneal anaesthesia lasting for up to 6 months; this makes toleration of contact lenses much easier during that period. Usually, however, the senile aphakic will eventually give up contact lenses and revert to spectacles (Ruben, 1982).

Lastly, it should be noted that a patient who has been markedly myopic prior to cataract removal may need no postoperative optical correction other than low-powered glasses for distance and reading.

In the author's experience, 98 per cent of patients who have had one cataract removed will return a second time. This must mean that the surgical procedure itself is innocuous and the results of such surgery of great value to the patient.

REFERENCES

Breslin P. P. (1973) *Int. Ophthalmol. Clin.* **13**, 215.

Cheng H. (1983) *J. R. Soc. Med.* **76**, 169.

Clayton R. M., Cuthbert R. J., Duffy J. et al. (1982) *Trans. Ophthalmol. Soc. UK.* **102**, 331.

Davidson S. I. (1984) Personal communication.

Eichenbaum D. N., Joffe N. S., Clayman H. M. et al. (1978). *Am. J. Ophthalmol.* **86**, 167.

Galin M. A., Dotson R. S., Obstraum S. A. et al. (1982) *Trans. Ophthalmol. Soc. UK.* **102**, 410.

Gilvarry A. and Eustace P. (1982) *Trans. Ophthalmol. Soc. UK.* **102**, 502.

Jacoby J. (1976) In: Duane T. D. (ed.) *Clinical Ophthalmology* Vol. 5, Chapter 1, Hagerstown Md., Harper & Row.

Jaffe N. S. (1981) *Cataract Surgery and its Complications.* St Louis, Mosby p. 576.

McLeod D., Restori M. and Wright J. E. (1977) *Br. J. Ophthalmol.* **61**, 437.

Ponte F., Anastasi M. and Lauricella M. (1981) In: Francois J. and Maumenee A. E. (eds) *Proceedings of 2nd International Congress on Cataract Surgery.* id Esente. 1, 35–37. Milan, Ghedini.

Rich W. (1982) *Trans. Ophthalmol. Soc. UK.* **102**, 407.

Rosen E. S. (1975) In: Bellows J. G. (ed.) *Cataract and Abnormalities of the Lens.* New York, Grune & Stratton, p. 469.

Ruben M. (1982) *Trans. Ophthalmol. Soc. UK.* **102**, 413.

Thompson C. R. S. and Harding G. F. A. (1977) *Doc. Ophthalmol.* **14**, p. 193–201.

8. INTRA-OCULAR PRESSURE AND GLAUCOMA
Calbert I. Phillips

AQUEOUS HUMOUR

The similarities between cerebrospinal fluid and aqueous humour are remarkable. Both are clear (in the eye, to achieve transparency) because of a very low cellular and protein content, although the plasma proteins are represented. Crystalloids (sodium, potassium, chloride, bicarbonate, etc.) are all in concentrations similar to those in plasma. In aqueous humour, ascorbate (vitamin C), pyruvate and lactate are present in higher concentrations than in plasma, probably in relation to metabolism of the lens.

There are analogies also in the production, circulation and draining of the two fluids (*Fig.* 8.1). Aqueous humour is, mainly, a secretion from the epithelium covering the highly vascular ciliary processes which are numerous finger-like projections from the surface of the ciliary body. Cerebrospinal fluid is secreted mainly by the choroid plexus of the lateral and fourth ventricles. Rather artificial analogies can be invented for the circulation: aqueous humour passes round the lens (much of it through the suspensory ligament) and through the pupil into the anterior chamber; perhaps the foramina in the roof of the fourth ventricle might correspond with the pupil.

Closer correspondence exists in the mechanism of drainage. Aqueous humour escapes from the eye through a very specialized tissue called the 'trabecular meshwork' at the base of the inner surface of the cornea: large droplets are engulfed by the deepest stratum, a single layer of endothelial cells, then pass across these cells to be 'excreted' into the canal of Schlemm. This mechanism is, surprisingly, pressure sensitive, i.e. increased outflow occurs when intra-ocular pressure rises. Arachnoid granulations in the intracranial venous sinuses probably serve a very similar mechanism for drainage of cerebrospinal fluid.

From the canal of Schlemm, aqueous humour drains into collector channels which pass outwards through the anterior sclera to join the subconjunctival veins.

A major function of aqueous humour is to nourish the lens. By means of a slight flow and diffusion posteriorly, it provides for the small

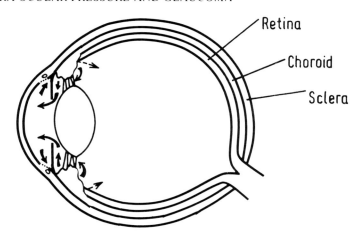

Retina

Choroid

Sclera

Fig. 8.1. Cross-section of eyeball. Aqueous humour is secreted by the ciliary epithelium behind the iris, flows through the pupil and into the angle of the anterior chamber. (This angle is between periphery of cornea and periphery of iris.) In the angle it passes through the trabecular meshwork (dotted lines) into the canal of Schlemm (small ovals). Thence it passes through collector channels into subconjunctival veins.

nutritional demands of the vitreous body. The normal intra-ocular pressure is 16 mmHg above atmospheric pressure, which maintains constancy of the size and shape of the eyeball and the position of the lens, which is important for the eye's optical function. There are small normal diurnal fluctuations in intra-ocular pressure.

INTRA-OCULAR PRESSURE AND ITS MEASUREMENT

Although the mean 'normal' intra-ocular pressure is about 16 mmHg, it does rise with increasing age.

The upper limit of normal is often taken as 24 mmHg, above which there is increasing danger of damage to the field of vision (*see below*): that figure is 3 standard deviations above the mean. A more stringent criterion of the upper limit would be 21 mmHg, which is 2 standard deviations above the mean.

Tonometry is to the ophthalmologist what sphygmomanometry is to other doctors—usually a routine part of most ophthalmic examinations, at least in patients over the age of 50 years. The applanation method is by far the commonest technique: 'applanation' because it depends on the pressure required to flatten a small standard area of the central cornea anaesthetized by a topical anaesthetic. A little fluorescein in an eyedrop introduced into the tears aids the estimation of the end-point: a thin film

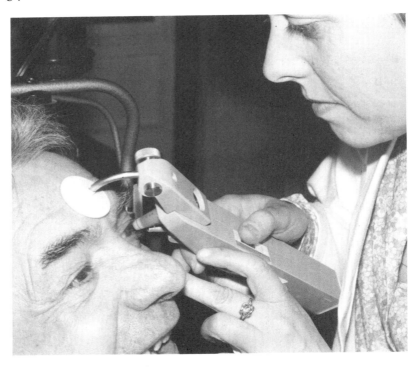

Fig. 8.2. Hand-held applanation tonometer.

of fluorescein-stained tears covers the surface of cornea (*see* *Fig.* 4.3).

A cylinder with a flat transparent surface at each end is used. It is carried on an arm which is spring-loaded to allow one flat end to be pressed gently on the corneal surface. The tonometrist looks through the other end, and through the microscope which is part of the standard slit-lamp microscope. The tonometrist can vary the pressure by a milled knob. He starts at a low level and gradually increases the pressure until the standard area of cornea is cleared of the tear film. The fluorescein makes the edge easily seen. The pressure is simply read off the graduations on the milled knob. The patient is hardly inconvenienced. For patients who cannot be moved to a slit-lamp microscope, a very accurate and convenient hand-held tonometer is available (*Fig.* 8.2).

THE GLAUCOMAS

These are a group of diseases whose common feature is a raised intra-ocular pressure. (There are exceptions to every rule: *see* 'low tension

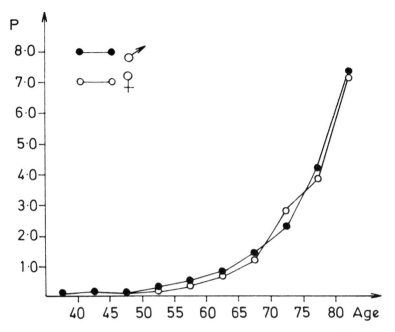

Fig. 8.3. The percentage (P) of sufferers from glaucoma in the population of Gothenburg, Sweden, rises from about 0·025 per cent before 45 years to more than 7 per cent by 80 years. (With grateful acknowledgements to *Acta Ophthalmologica, Copenhagen* Popovic, 1982.)

glaucoma' *below.*) Another common feature is that all are due to impaired drainage of aqueous humour, although the mechanism is different in different diseases. Abnormally high production of aqueous humour is never a cause of glaucoma. A great deal is known about the causes of the glaucomas so that the term 'primary glaucoma', still sometimes applied to open-angle and angle-closure (= closed-angle) glaucoma, need no longer be used. A better case can be made out for retaining the term 'secondary glaucomas' for steroid- and lens-induced, iridocyclitic, and other glaucomas (*see below*).

Epidemiology of Open-angle and Angle-closure Glaucoma

A recent survey of the population of Gothenburg, Sweden (Popovic, 1982), has confirmed similar previous observations in other countries on the prevalence of glaucoma (*Fig.* 8.3). It is very low before the fourth decade (about 0·025 per cent) but rises exponentially thereafter to reach over 7 per cent in the eighth. First degree relatives (children, siblings and parents) can be expected to suffer a prevalence of around three times that in the general population, an indication in favour of a screening programme for that group at least.

Around one-third of the total glaucoma population have the angle-closure type. Almost all the others have the open-angle (chronic simple) variety, so that the remainder, some of which are briefly mentioned in this chapter, constitute a very small, though important, minority.

Open-angle (Chronic Simple) Glaucoma (OAG/CSG)

OAG/CSG is due to an inherited defect in the function of the endothelial layer of the trabecular meshwork which is responsible for passing aqueous humour into the canal of Schlemm. Normally, this function becomes less efficient with age, as also does the production of aqueous humour; a slight imbalance causes the gradual rise of normal intra-ocular pressure with age. However, in patients with OAG this deterioration in outflow is much more marked than usual, but it is very likely that, even when these patients were young, their intra-ocular pressure was higher than the average for their age group. The exact metabolic abnormality is not known. The term 'open-angle' is used to emphasize the absence of the hallmark of 'angle-closure' glaucoma, viz. in the latter disease occlusion of the trabecular meshwork by the periphery of the iris.

Clinical Features: At first, even when the pressure is above, say, 24 mmHg (the field-losing threshold), no disturbance of function occurs, i.e. there are no symptoms. At this stage some prefer the diagnosis 'ocular hypertension' rather than OAG. Gonioscopy must be done at the first visit to establish that the periphery of the iris is not occluding the trabecular meshwork.

As a result of the raised intra-ocular pressure, the optic disc gradually develops pathological cupping (*Fig.* 8.4), along with a very typical pattern of field loss. There are two schools of thought on the pathological process involved in cupping of the optic disc. The mechanists believe that the raised pressure picks out the softest part of the wall of the eyeball and pushes it mechanically outwards, gradually breaking or stretching the nerve fibres as they leave the retina to form the optic nerve. The more popular vascular school believes that the nerve fibres suffer ischaemic necrosis slowly because the raised intra-ocular pressure cuts off their blood supply. The diameter of the cup, which is visible in most normal optic discs, can be up to two-thirds of the diameter of the optic disc and still be considered normal. In estimating the cup-to-disc ratio, it is better to use the vertical meridian than the horizontal, but the difference is small. When the cup : disc ratio reaches 3 : 4 or more, the diagnosis of glaucoma is very likely. Cup : disc ratios between 2 : 3 and 3 : 4 induce in the observer a glaucoma neurosis: he becomes aware of the dilemma—should he or should he not do tonometry, fields of vision and gonioscopy? A cup : disc ratio of less than 2 : 3 (e.g. 1 : 2, 1 : 3, 1 : 4) is very probably 'safe'.

PLATE I

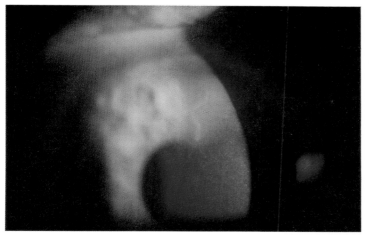

Sodium fluorescein staining of a dendritic ulcer (6 o'clock).

PLATE II

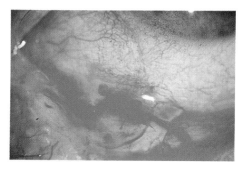

1. Stringy discharge staining with Rose Bengal, visible without biomicroscopy.

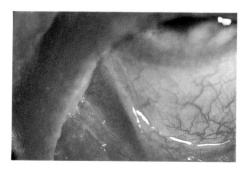

2. Symblepharon—contracture of the epithelium and subepithelial tissues.

PLATE III

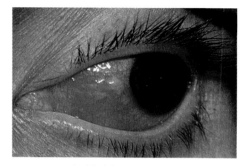

1. Nodules in scleritis.

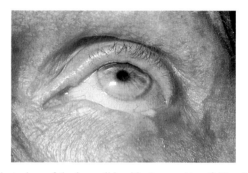

2. Rodent ulcer of the lower lid, with recurrent 'cyst'-like chalazia.

PLATE IV

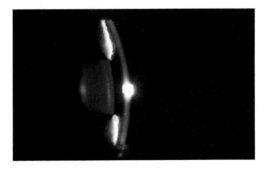

Slit lamp view of posterior subcapsular opacity. Central bright spot is beam on cornea, upper and lower bright spots are iris, and lens with bright spot (opacity) is to the right.

PLATE V

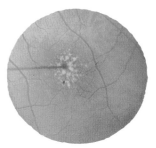

1. Drusen of Bruch's Membrane. This the right macula of a patient of 60, showing macular drusen. The visual acuity of this eye is 6/6.

2. Atrophy of Retinal Pigment Epithelium. This is the right eye of a patient with a visual acuity of 6/18 showing drusen, but in addition areas of macular retinal pigment epithelial atrophy. There is no serous detachment. No treatment is possible for this lesion.

PLATE VI

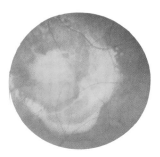

1. Disciform Macular Degeneration. This is the macula of a patient with very poor central vision, showing an elevated macular disciform lesion. There is central sub-retinal neovascular tissue and surrounding sub-retinal exudates. No treatment is possible at this advanced stage of macular degeneration.

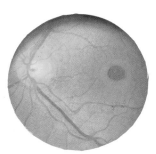

2. Macular Hole. This is the left macula of a 75-year-old patient complaining of sudden loss of central vision. It shows a full thickness macular hole, for which no treatment is possible.

PLATE VII

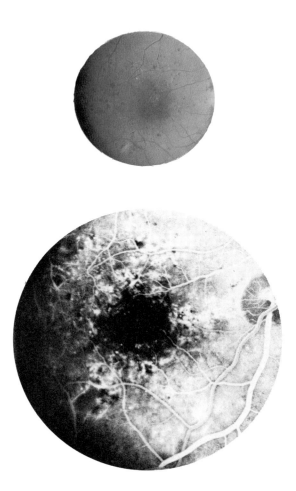

Background Retinopathy with early Macular Involvement. Maturity onset diabetes of 18 months' duration. Many microaneurysms and small haemorrhages, which show dye leakage. One soft exudate below macula with underlying area of capillary non-perfusion. Visual acuity 6/9.

PLATE VIII

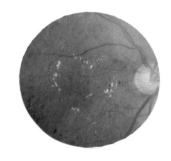

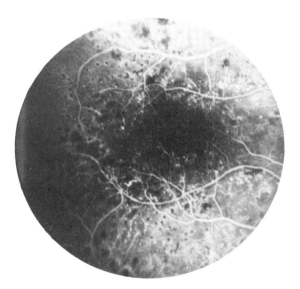

Focal Maculopathy. Maturity onset diabetes of 17 years' duration. Gradual drop in visual acuities. Groups of microaneurysms, small haemorrhages, hard exudates in macular area, and a few soft exudates. Marks of laser photocoagulation can be seen around the macular area especially on the fluoresein angiogram.

PLATE IX

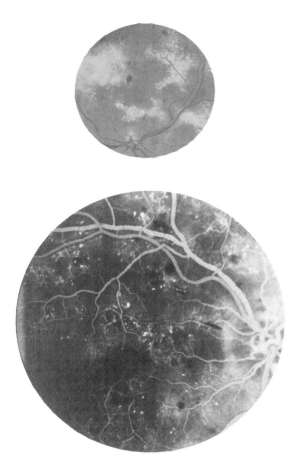

Exudative Maculopathy. Recently diagnosed maturity onset diabetes. Vision severely diminished in both eyes due to extensive exudative maculopathy. Large confluent plaques of hard exudate. Angiogram shows many microaneurysms and small vessel abnormalities, with dye leakage.

PLATE X

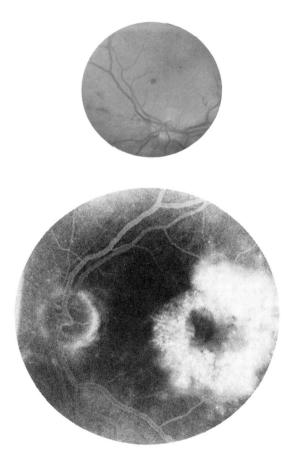

Cystoid Maculopathy. Maturity onset diabetes of 13 years' duration. Gradual decline in vision in right eye due to cystoid maculopathy. Macula shows signs of background retinopathy, but not grossly abnormal. Angiogram shows marked cystoid macular oedema. Visual acuity 6/18.

PLATE XI

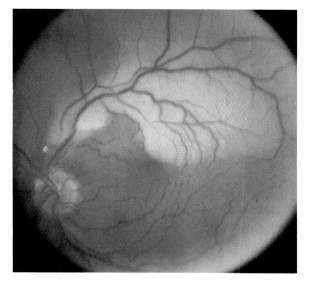

1. Occlusion by embolus (arrowed) of upper temporal arteriole.

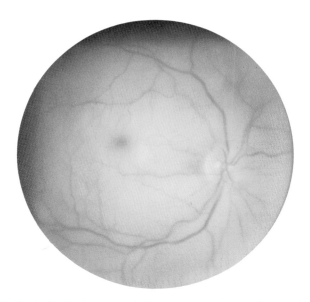

2. Cortical retinal artery occlusion—cherry red spot at the macula.

PLATE XII

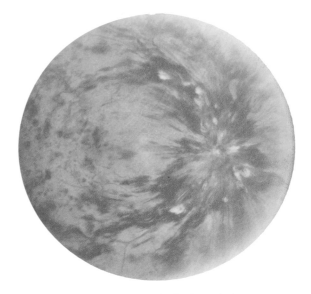

1. Recent central retinal vein occlusion.

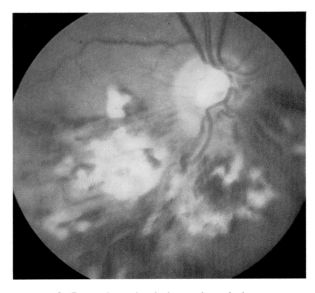

2. Recent lower hemisphere vein occlusion.

PLATE XIII

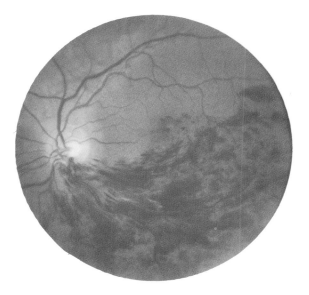

Inferior temporal vein occlusion.

PLATE XIV

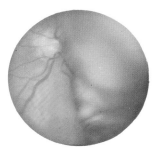

1. Solid retinal detachment showing raised and irregular surface.

2. Non-solid retinal detachment showing grey areas of separated retina (bottom right, top left) and normal intervening flat retina.

PLATE XV

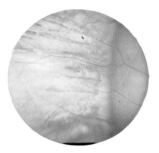

1. Regular edge between re-attached indented retina on the left and atrophic retina to the right.

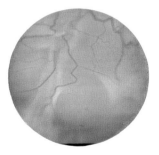

2. Traction bands maintaining detachment.

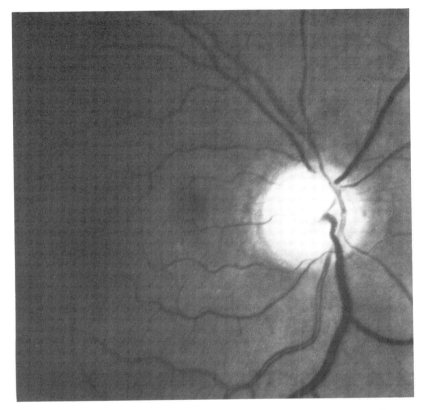

Fig. 8.4. Pathological cupping. The disc is pale. Raised intra-ocular pressure has pushed the disc posteriorly leaving a sharp edge: note how the retinal blood vessels angulate sharply at the disc edge and the large ones superiorly disappear under the overhanging edge of the disc.

Although the disease is bilateral, one eye is quite often affected before, or to a greater extent than the other. Accordingly, if the ophthalmoscopist can detect any difference between the right and left cup : disc ratios in a patient, even if both are less than 2 : 3, the diagnosis of OAG should be suspected.

The most vulnerable nerve fibres lie at the lower margin of the disc, hence the typical pattern of early field loss (*Fig.* 8.5). Gradually other fibres are affected each time the pressure rises above the field-losing level, with a characteristic progression of field loss until there remains only a tube-field (or tunnel vision) and even that is eventually engulfed in the rising tide of blindness (*Fig.* 8.6).

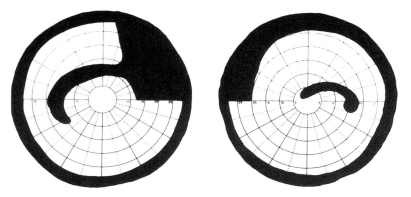

Fig. 8.5. The right field shows an 'arcuate' scotoma arching nasally from the blind spot. The left field loss is more advanced with larger 'basal step'.

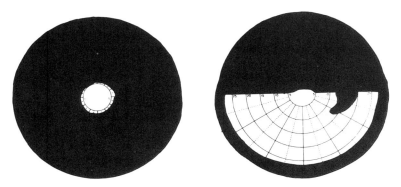

Fig. 8.6. The right upper half field has disappeared. The left eye retains only a small central area of vision—'tube field' or 'tunnel vision'.

Early Diagnosis: The disease may be well advanced with considerable field loss before the patient notices any real disability, especially if one eye is more affected than the other. The visual acuity usually remains good until late in the disease. That applies particularly to the elderly. Accordingly the refractionist, ophthalmologist or optician, seeing the presbyope regularly every few years to increase the strength of his reading spectacles, must examine the optic discs and record the (vertical) cup : disc ratio at each attendance. Ophthalmoscopy is part of any full general medical examination, so that the general practitioner, the geriatrician, and all physicians but especially the neurologist, must 'screen' the optic discs of his population for glaucomatous changes. That criterion is better than tonometry, which is of course the next stage in the assessment, along with plotting of the fields of vision.

Low-tension Glaucoma is a quite extraordinary and fascinating disease, constituting 2 or 3 per cent of all OAGs. The disease is exactly like OAG, with pathological cupping and very slowly increasing field loss, but the intra-ocular pressure is normal! The cause is unknown: a commonly used rationalization may have some truth, viz. that the optic disc or its blood supply in these particular patients cannot withstand even the normal intra-ocular pressure.

Treatment is aimed at reducing the intra-ocular pressure, even in 'low-tension' glaucoma; medical treatment is preferable, but drainage operations are sometimes necessary.

The first line of defence is Timoptol (timolol) eye drops 0·25 or 0·5 per cent, twice or once daily. This beta-1 and beta-2 blocking drug penetrates into the eye, probably through the cornea, and reduces pressure by reducing the production of aqueous humour. Perhaps rather surprisingly, there is no evidence of any tendency to produce cataract. Some systemic absorption occurs to reduce pulse rate by about 10 per cent, to reduce blood pressure, and to produce all the other side-effects of beta blockers. Accordingly, these drops should be used with great caution, if at all, in patients with bradycardia or cardiac decompensation, and asthma/chronic bronchitis/emphysema. Conversely, the ophthalmologist must not be misled by an unexpectedly low intra-ocular pressure in an obviously glaucomatous patient who is receiving a beta-blocking drug orally for, say, vascular hypertension, because that route of administration will cause a fall in intra-ocular pressure.

Rather paradoxically, adrenaline eye drops also cause a fall in intra-ocular pressure, mainly by increasing outflow of aqueous humour. This drug of course also dilates the pupil and, by systemic absorption, may produce general adrenergic stimulation. Because of the danger of angle-closure glaucoma which can be precipitated by mydriasis (*see below*), this drug should never be used in that disease, unless iridectomy or a drainage operation have already been done.

Pilocarpine 0·5—4 per cent eye drops every 3, 4 or 6 hours are the traditional treatment, and are often combined with one of the above drugs. This reduces pressure in OAG by a direct effect on the muscle cells of the ciliary body which, when they contract, pull on the trabecular meshwork and that—somehow—improves the outflow of aqueous humour. An unfortunate side-effect is contraction of the sphincter muscle of the pupil with miosis, which cuts down the light entering the eye and so 'darkens' the vision. (*See* mechanism of action of pilocarpine in angle-closure glaucoma *below.*)

Dilute concentrations (0·12 or 0·06 per cent) of Phospholine Iodide (ecothiopate iodide), a very powerful cholinergic drug, are sometimes used. Depression of serum pseudocholinesterase will endanger the anaesthetized patient if the muscle-relaxant succinylcholine is used.

Systemic drugs, even long-term, may be used especially if there is a special reason for avoiding drainage operations. Carbonic anhydrase inhibitors reduce the amount of bicarbonate secreted into the aqueous humour, and also the water necessary to carry it, and so cut down the volume of aqueous humour produced. Tablets of acetazolamide (Diamox) 250 mg twice daily (or in 'Sustets', enteric coated capsules of 500 mg once daily), along with potassium bicarbonate 600 mg daily to counteract the increased urinary loss of potassium, are usually prescribed. Dichlorphenamide (Daranide) 60 mg twice daily may be substituted for acetazolamide. I advise almost all patients who are taking tablets of any kind to take them in the middle of a meal, to avoid the discomfort and possible danger of delayed transit at a narrow point in the oesophagus—a chemical oesophagitis or actual oesophageal 'burn' may occur.

The glaucomatous patient attends the ophthalmologist for his lifetime, mainly to have the visual fields plotted, but of course tonometry is also important. A drainage operation is indicated when field loss continues and/or the raised pressure is not controlled on maximum tolerable medical treatment. The common property of almost all drainage operations is to provide aqueous humour with a route of escape through the corneo-scleral junction into the subconjunctival space. The most commonly performed operation at present, trabeculectomy, has fewer complications than previous ones and many surgeons intervene at an earlier stage in the disease process than in the days of trephines, sclerectomies and iris inclusions: that would apply particularly in the elderly whose compliance with medical treatment regimens is, understandably, often inefficient.

In spite of all these treatments, OAG remains a common cause of blindness.

Steroid Glaucoma is very like OAG in every way. Within 3–6 weeks of starting steroid eye drops, about 10 per cent of the population will develop a raised pressure, although some steroids (e.g. clobetasone) are less glaucomatogenic than others (e.g. dexamethasone). That 10 per cent represents the proportion of the population who have, or are going to have OAG, plus those who have inherited the predisposition but would not have ever developed the disease. Patients are on record, for example in the archives of the medical defence societies, who have gone blind from glaucoma due to steroid eye drops prescribed for relatively trivial 'sore eyes' or 'chronic conjunctivitis'. Another situation in which steroids are dangerous is the red eye when the diagnosis of dendritic ulcer (due to the herpes virus) has been missed—disastrous spread of infection (with improvement in symptoms) occurs. Accordingly many eye specialists advocate that steroid eye drops, alone or in combination with

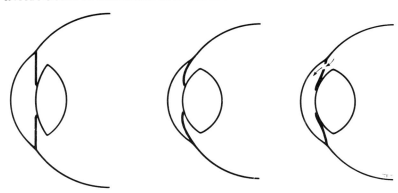

Fig. 8.7. Diagrams of anterior segments of eyeballs. The left diagram represents the configuration of a normal eye, or an eye with open-angle glaucoma. The centre diagram shows an eye predisposed to angle closure glaucoma: the shallow anterior chamber and narrow angle result from an axially thick lens, anteriorly placed, and small diameter cornea; aqueous humour meets resistance at the pupil, hence ballooning of the iris which narrows the angle even more. The right diagram shows how peripheral iridectomy, surgical or laser-produced, will eliminate the ballooning of iris and will open the angle considerably.

antibiotics, etc., should only be used under close ophthalmological supervision.

Angle-closure (Closed-angle) Glaucoma (ACG/CAG)

ACG/CAG has a completely different mechanism (*Fig.* 8.7). The patient inherits a small eyeball, which may also be hypermetropic. Nature attempts to compensate optically for this by producing a more powerful lens in the eye, to try to bring rays of light to a focus in a shorter distance; for similar optical reasons the whole lens is probably positioned a little more anteriorly in the eyeball. A 'more powerful lens' implies a steeper curvature of its surfaces, and therefore a greater axial thickness. Associated with the small overall size of the eyeball is a small diameter cornea. This may be obvious to the observer if he holds the lids apart and inspects the eyeball closely—compare the larger-than-normal myopic eye which never suffers ACG.

The effect of these abnormalities is that the pupil is 'pushed' forwards to a plane more anterior than the periphery of the iris. The 'eclipse test' may demonstrate this anatomical peculiarity: a narrow torch light is shone from the temporal side, along a plane passing through the mid-iris and a note is made whether the iris is in shadow on the nasal side.

There are three results from the anterior position of the pupil:
1. The anterior chamber is shallower than usual, as implied above;

2. The angle of the anterior chamber is necessarily narrow, which is aggravated, because—
3. Aqueous humour meets more than usual resistance at the pupil, so that the pressure difference between the back and front of the iris is greater than usual and so the iris balloons forwards (*iris bombe*)— rather like a spinnaker in the breeze, to use an exaggerated analogy.

   On that background, the following property of the lens in all eyes becomes potentially disastrous;
4. The lens goes on increasing in size, including axial thickness, throughout life.

In these small predisposed eyes, the pupil is gradually pushed forwards, narrowing the angle and increasing the resistance at the pupil to the passage of aqueous humour which causes more ballooning of the iris to narrow the angle even more. One of two things then happen. The more dramatic is sudden closure of the angle all round, i.e. occlusion of the whole trabecular meshwork by the periphery of the iris. Within a few hours the intra-ocular pressure rises almost to equal the diastolic blood pressure (60 mmHg) with severe pain, sometimes enough to cause vomiting, severe redness and corneal oedema. The cornea becomes rather like frosted glass which reduces the patient's visual acuity and obscures the observer's view of the shallow anterior chamber and the typically vertically oval pupil. The name for this disease was 'acute congestive glaucoma'. The patient should be asked to look down and the stony hardness and tenderness of the eye noted when it is tested for fluctuation through the upper lid. Inspection of the fellow eye will reveal the anatomical predisposition; having come from the same factory it is predisposed to the same disease. Indeed the acute disease is sometimes bilateral.

The less dramatic outcome, in about one-third of cases, depends on the fact that the upper angle is narrower than the lower. The angle often closes gradually from above downwards with a gradually rising pressure to produce pathological cupping and field loss, i.e. a disease very like OAG but for the anatomical state of the anterior chamber and, in particular, the high proportion of the trabecular meshwork occluded by peripheral iris.

Gonioscopy: A special contact lens (gonioscope) has to be used to allow the observer to see the angle of the anterior chamber, with magnification by the slit-lamp microscope (*Fig.* 8.8). This examination is essential for the differentiation of open-angle from angle-closure glaucoma.

Treatment: The most important treatment of the patient with acute (or chronic) ACG is actually to instil pilocarpine 0·5 per cent immediately into the *fellow* eye and every 3 hours, to cause miosis (and pull the periphery of the iris away from the trabecular meshwork), along with

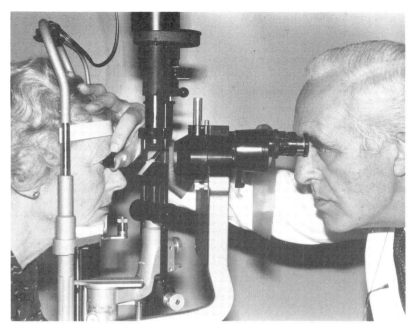

Fig. 8.8. Gonioscopy. The essential part is a contact lens to allow rays of light coming from the angle of the anterior chamber to avoid total internal reflection at the cornea-air interface. A mirror in the gonioscope reflects the rays of light forwards into the microscope to give the observer a magnified view of the angle of the anterior chamber.

Timoptol 0·5 per cent twice daily, to reduce the *iris bombe* until prophylactic peripheral iridectomy or laser iridotomy can be done; otherwise acute ACG is liable to occur at any time. Pilocarpine 2 per cent every 15 minutes to the eye with acute ACG may help, but *urgent referral to an ophthalmic surgeon within a few hours* is essential because the sooner iridectomy or (if the trabecular meshwork is likely to be permanently totally occluded) a drainage operation is done, the better is the prognosis for a good visual result—after the pre-operative preliminary of intravenous hypertonic mannitol and/or acetazolamide (Diamox) is given to reduce intra-ocular pressure to normal (*Fig.* 8.7).

The rationale of iridectomy or laser iridotomy is to allow aqueous to by-pass the resisting pupil, and collapse the *iris bombe*, thereby reducing the narrowness of the angle. That is enough to prevent ACG during any patient's lifetime, although of course the angle does remain narrow and indeed becomes increasingly narrow as the lens continues to grow in size.

Lens-induced Glaucoma

A densely cataractous lens, usually if it has been in that state for many years, may become hypermature and swollen ('intumescent') to make the anterior chamber extremely shallow and drive the periphery of the iris on to the trabecular meshwork—with an acute rise in pressure, just as in ACG. The elderly are the most at risk from this sort of glaucoma. Treatment is emergency cataract extraction after reduction of intraocular pressure by intravenous hypertonic mannitol with or without acetazolamide (Diamox).

There are two other ways by which a hypermature cataract can produce a rather acute glaucoma. Such a lens may break up and the lens matter silts up the trabecular meshwork. Also, degenerating, even liquefied, lens products may cause an inflammation of the iris and ciliary body (toxic iridocyclitis) from which the inflammatory exudate silts up the trabecular meshwork. Surgical removal of the lens matter is indicated in both cases. This 'silting up' is also the mechanism of glaucoma when it occurs as a complication of iridocyclitis, but that is very uncommon in the elderly, unless there have been episodes in earlier life.

REFERENCE
Popovič V. (1982) *Acta Ophthalmol. (Copenh.)* **60**, 745.

9. MACULAR DEGENERATION
J. S. Shilling

Macular degeneration is a very important cause of visual loss in the elderly. Patients with disease of the macula represent a significant number of those presenting to ophthalmic clinics with visual deterioration (*see* Chapter 1). Until recently there has been very little, if any, chance of restoring the vision in this group of patients by any form of therapy, but with the development of lasers, there is hope for some with specific types of degeneration. This chapter describes the symptoms and signs commonly encountered in macular disease and reviews the present status of treatment for these conditions.

SYMPTOMS

The commonest symptom of macular disease is blurred central vision. Patients complain of difficulty with reading and seeing fine detail and this may progress to formation of a dense central scotoma in some patients. In the early phases other symptoms are noticed, particularly metamorphopsia (visual distortion). This is usually recognized as irregularities and bending of straight lines. These symptoms may occur suddenly and, with progression of the degeneration, become more troublesome. Patients may also notice a change in image size; this is usually a minification of the image (micropsia). Both these preceding symptoms are due to abnormal orientation of the macular receptors. Changes in the perception of colour (dischromatopsia) and abnormal light sensations are also often reported.

PHYSICAL SIGNS

The physical signs of macular degeneration are only visible after full dilatation of the pupil with mydriatic drops. It is not possible to examine the macula properly in the undilated state, and it is incorrect to make any assessment of the macula without dilatation. The macula may be examined by direct ophthalmoscopy, but this gives merely a monocular view. Full assessment must include examination of the macula with either a contact lens or a Hruby lens attached to the examining slit-lamp

95

microscope. Only with the latter instrument is it possible to identify subtle macular changes.

Examination of the macula in an elderly patient may reveal 'normal' ageing changes and in addition, various degenerative changes may also be observed. The normal ageing changes consist of thinning of the retinal pigment epithelium, recognized as a change in the colour of the retina, and the presence of colloid bodies which are seen as pale circumscribed lesions at the posterior pole of the eye (*Plate V 1*). These changes may not affect vision although sometimes appearing quite extensive, and it is important that other causes of visual loss should be considered when a patient presents with visual loss and these abnormalities, because other pathologies may be present simultaneously, for example, cataract, glaucoma, or neurological disease. When the visual acuity drops due to macular disease, other physical signs appear in addition to the above. There may be extensive loss of the retinal pigment epithelium and of the small choroidal capillaries. This leads to an atrophic appearance, which at its most extreme is described as central areolar choroidal atrophy (*Plate V 2*). This condition is slowly progressive, may involve one or both eyes and is not amenable to any specific therapy. Various drug therapies have been tried, but there is no good evidence that any medication is effective in slowing down or reversing the macular atrophy. Visual loss in this type of degeneration is usually slowly progressive, but patients may retain some central vision for a long time. Sarks (1976) has described the ageing changes in a large clinico-pathological study. She has defined the stages of senile changes by looking at macular histology, in eyes which had been previously examined clinically and by retinal photography.

DISCIFORM MACULAR DEGENERATION

The most severe type of senile macular degeneration is that termed 'disciform'. In this condition, in which there may be sudden central visual loss, examination reveals a serous detachment of the neuroretina due to a sub-retinal neovascular membrane growing from the choroidal circulation through a dehiscence in Bruch's membrane. The neovascular membrane is best shown by fluorescein angiography. This technique reveals the sub-retinal new vessels which leak fluorescein profusely because of their loose capillary endothelial junctions. It is abnormal leakage of fluid from these blood vessels that causes the serous detachment of the macular retina and subsequent visual deterioration (*Plate VI 1*). Gass (1967) describes the abnormalities in detail.

It is in this type of macular degeneration that laser photocoagulation has found a place. It is possible by using argon or krypton laser applications to destroy sub-retinal neovascular tissue with subsequent flattening of the retina. Unfortunately this treatment is not applicable to all patients with disciform macular degeneration. The new vessels may grow in an area away from the fovea or may originate from the sub-foveal region. Although technically possible, destruction of new vessels beneath the fovea results in gross atrophy of the foveal area and therefore permanent loss of vision. Treatment of membranes is therefore only possible if the membrane has originated outside and not extended into the immediate sub-foveal region. The position of the membrane as defined by fluorescein angiography identifies those patients with extra-foveal neovascular tissue for which photocoagulation is then appropriate. It is important that the ophthalmologist recognizes the principle of treatment of neovascular membranes. Total destruction of the membranes by photocoagulation is essential because regrowth of tissue will otherwise occur, often subsequently involving the sub-foveal area with permanent loss of vision. Various controlled studies performed to evaluate the efficacy of this treatment have shown benefit from photocoagulation therapy in those disciform lesions lying away from the fovea (American Macular Study Group, 1982; Moorfields Macular Study Group, 1982 a). The exact criteria for treatment vary in different centres, but it is usually recognized that a sub-retinal membrane lying more than 200 μm from the foveola may be within the therapeutic range.

Treatment of disciform macular degeneration is now a recognized ophthalmological emergency, because the growth of a new vessel membrane may be rapid. Although patients with early symptoms may have a membrane lying eccentric to the fovea, this may grow rapidly and involve the foveal area within a few days. Patients presenting with visual distortion or other symptoms of early macular degeneration should be referred urgently for fluorescein angiography and assessment for laser photocoagulation. Ideally a period of not more than twenty-four hours should elapse between diagnosis, fluorescein angiography, and laser treatment. It may be difficult to achieve this for logistical reasons, but units performing the treatment must try to arrange their services as efficiently as possible.

Prognosis of Disciform Macular Degeneration

Patients presenting with a disciform macular lesion in one eye are at risk of a similar occurrence in the second eye. It has been calculated that there is a 10–12 per cent chance per year of involvement of the second eye (Teeters and Bird, 1973a and b; Grey et al., 1979). It is therefore very important that this group of patients is told to report urgently if vision in their second eye should change, so that early investigation and treatment may be instituted. Unfortunately, following laser photocoagulation of a disciform lesion, there is still a risk of further disciform lesions developing in the treated eye. This again has been calculated to be approximately 10–12 per cent per year.

OTHER MACULAR DISORDERS IN THE ELDERLY

Macular atrophy and disciform macular degeneration are unquestionably the commonest disorders in the elderly, but other conditions do occur.

Avascular Retinal Pigment Epithelial Detachment

Avascular retinal pigment epithelial detachment is another type of process at the macula in senile eyes. The patient presents with some visual loss, and an elevation of the macula is found. This elevation occurs at the level of the retinal pigment epithelium, which separates from Bruch's membrane. The lesion has a greyish colour, and is associated with drusen of Bruch's membrane. There is little serous detachment of the neuro-retina. Fluorescein demonstrates slow filling of the detached area, but no evidence of neovascularization.

The pigment epithelial detachment may remain unchanged for many months, but may develop into a disciform lesion later, or sometimes resolves spontaneously.

Photocoagulation was tried and although some good results were obtained, neovascularization following treatment occurred. A controlled trial of argon laser treatment was instituted but was aborted because treatment was found to cause a higher incidence of disciform development than occurred spontaneously. These lesions are therefore now not treated (Moorfields Macular Study Group, 1982b).

Myopic Macular Degeneration

Patients with high myopia are liable to lose central vision because of macular disease. This may occur at any age, but elderly subjects are not excluded (see Chapter 1). Macular haemorrhage is common, and central visual loss is the result. The haemorrhage is usually due to a myopic variety of disciform degeneration, for which the eponymous term 'Foster-Fuch's fleck' is used. These lesions are usually pigmented and small by comparison with other disciform lesions. They may be beneath the fovea, when no treatment is possible; occasionally they are not, and laser treatment is then sometimes useful. The prognosis for central vision is not so poor in this special group of patients.

Macular Hole

The occurrence of a full thickness hole at the macular is an important cause of visual loss in the elderly. This lesion presents with visual distortion, followed by loss of central visual acuity; examination shows a circular hole at the macula through which the underlying retinal pigment epithelium is visible (Plate VI 2). This lesion is untreatable and results in a permanent central visual loss. Patients with a macular hole in one eye have a small risk of a similar lesion developing in the second eye (Aaberg et al., 1970).

Pre-retinal Macular Traction Membrane

The formation of a traction membrane at the macula is a common macular abnormality in the elderly. This lesion presents with distortion of vision and some central visual loss. Examination of the macula shows irregularity of the retina with traction lines emanating from an area of pre-retinal fibro-glial tissue. This lesion is often associated with a detachment of the posterior vitreous; sometimes peripheral retinal holes or retinal detachment occur simultaneously. Visual loss with a macular traction membrane is not usually extreme, although severe macular oedema or a traction macular detachment may occur in which case the visual acuity drops precipitously (Wise, 1975). Treatment for this condition is usually conservative in the elderly. It is possible to remove a traction membrane by a vitrectomy/membranectomy operation; some good results have been reported (Michels, 1981). However, visual acuity in the elderly patient is not usually sufficiently damaged to warrant this extensive surgery. Usually patients with this condition have a normal fellow eye which is at very little risk of a similar condition and therefore surgery is not usually carried out.

Retinal Vascular Disease (*see* Chapter 11)

Macular damage due to retinal vascular disease may occur in the elderly but is not specific to this age group. Occlusion of retinal veins, either of the central vein or of its branches may occur particularly in hypertensive and atherosclerotic patients. These may present with loss of central visual acuity due to macular haemorrhage, macular oedema, ischaemia of the macula, or sometimes a pre-retinal traction membrane associated with the vascular disease. Photocoagulation is sometimes used for some of the complications of these vascular conditions.

Retinal artery occlusion may also affect the macula. Central retinal artery occlusion causes very severe visual loss and usually no perception of light, but branch artery occlusions may effect small areas of retina. A macular arteriolar blockage can be difficult to differentiate from other causes of central loss. These arteriolar diseases often have an embolic basis, and their identification therefore leads to systemic vascular investigations and possibly specific therapy to prevent other embolic phenomena.

GENERAL MANAGEMENT OF MACULAR DEGENERATION

There has been considerable advance in the treatment of macular degeneration during the last few years. However, many patients with macular degeneration of various types lose normal central vision permanently. It is important that these patients receive supportive measures in their visual loss. The use of low vision aids may be extremely helpful, even if visual acuity is quite poor. Although normal acuity cannot be restored, it is often possible with special magnifying aids for these people to retain some visual independence, enabling them to read important documents for near and using telescopic aids for distance. It is important to stress to these patients that total visual loss does not occur from macular degeneration and that the peripheral visual field, giving them social independence, will be retained permanently.

Blind or partial sight registration enables patients to obtain social services and other advantages only available to blind people and it is important that the social services take a full part in the rehabilitation of patients with the crippling retinal macular diseases (*see* Chapter 15).

REFERENCES

Aaberg T. M., Blair C. J., Gass J. D. M. (1970) *Am. J. Ophthalmol.* **69**, 555–562.
American Macular Study Group (1982) *Arch. Ophthalmol.* **100**, 912–918.
Gass J. D. M. (1967) *Am. J. Ophthalmol.* **63**, 617–660.
Grey R. H. B., Bird A. C., Chisholm I. H. (1979) *Br. J. Ophthalmol.* **63**, 85–89.
Michels R. G. (1981) *Ophthalmol.* **81**, No. 11, 1384–1388.
Moorfields Macular Study Group (1982a) *Br. J. Ophthalmol.* **66**, 745–753.
Moorfields Macular Study Group (1982b) *Br. J. Ophthalmol.* **66**, 1–16.
Sarks S. H. (1976) *Br. J. Ophthalmol.* **60**, 324–341.
Teeters V. W. and Bird A. C. (1973a) *Am. J. Ophthalmol.* **75**, 53–65.
Teeters V. W. and Bird A. C. (1973b) *Am. J. Ophthalmol.* **76**, 1–18.
Wise G. N. (1975) *Am. J. Ophthalmol.* **79**, 349–357.

10. DIABETIC RETINOPATHY
H. Kennedy and F. I. Caird

Epidemiological studies of diabetic retinopathy show that it is a not uncommon problem in the elderly, causing 7 per cent of blindness registrations over the age of 65 (*see* Chapter 1). The numbers of patients with other ocular diseases (including these when they occur in diabetics) so greatly increase with age that diabetic retinopathy is relatively less important in the elderly than in the young. Yet approximately half of all patients blind from diabetic retinopathy are over 70 years old (Committee on Blindness, 1970).

It is now possible, by good supervision of the diabetes and of the visual state by physician and ophthalmologist together, and early and adequate treatment by photocoagulation where indicated, to prevent blindness in a large proportion of sufferers from retinopathy. Appropriate referral by the physician to the ophthalmologist is the most important part of a system of ocular care for diabetics of any age.

INCIDENCE

Diabetic retinopathy is a complication of the diabetic state, and so occurs to a greater or lesser degree in all forms of diabetes of whatever aetiology. In this context, any attempt at classification of types of diabetes seems to be irrelevant to the problem, in old age at least. There is some evidence—the certainty remains in doubt—that retinopathy is negatively associated with the genetically determined state of chlorpropamide-alcohol flushing (Leslie et al., 1979). Whatever the truth of this may be, there are certainly many both insulin requiring and non-insulin requiring elderly diabetics with retinopathy.

The occurrence of diabetic retinopathy, both with and without symptoms, is critically related to the age at onset of the disease and its duration, and to its degree of metabolic control. The chances of its developing are of the same order in elderly patients as in younger. Approximately 50 per cent of patients of all ages have retinopathy after 15 years of diabetes, but in the elderly it may develop more rapidly in the earlier years (Burditt et al., 1968; Pirart, 1977). There is evidence that control in the first few years of diabetes is especially important in determining the occurrence of diabetic retinopathy at a later date; this applies to patients with onset after as well as before the age of 60 (Constam, 1965; Caird et al., 1969).

The pattern of retinal involvement in diabetic retinopathy is different in elderly patients from that seen in middle age or younger. So-called 'malignant' or proliferative retinopathy, with the high risk features of new vessel formation, venous disease, and vitreous haemorrhage—the common precipitants of blindness in younger patients—are rarely encountered in patients over 70 (see Caird, 1982). The predominant pathology in the retina is exudative in type, and in so far as the macula is involved visual impairment or blindness frequently result. The rate of progression of retinopathy, and so the chances of blindness, rise with age, so that in patients with retinopathy and initially good vision the chances of blindness are about six times greater in the elderly than in the young (see Caird et al., 1969). In patients over the age of 60 years when their diabetes is diagnosed, 38 per cent of those with background retinopathy will suffer from moderate to severe visual loss within five years (Caird, 1965). In the great majority maculopathy is the cause.

EXAMINATION

About 10 per cent of patients with diabetes presenting in old age have retinopathy at the time of diagnosis (Soler et al., 1969), so that regular examination of the eyes is necessary from the time of first recognition of diabetes. Because of the large numbers involved, the proper place for this follow-up is at the diabetic clinic, by physicians experienced in fundoscopy in diabetes. Those patients found to have more than a minimal degree of retinopathy, or who complain of a drop in visual acuity, should be referred to the ophthalmologist for further investigation and follow-up by him as necessary.

Assessment of these patients by the ophthalmologist includes the recording of corrected visual acuities, ophthalmoscopy by both direct and indirect methods, and slit-lamp examination with the fundus contact lens. Periodic colour fundus photography is also of value; the photographs provide a permanent record for the purposes of comparison with later appearances, and a further advantage is that, while individual lesions in the fundus can be missed by experienced observers, this is less likely when colour photographs are projected onto a screen.

Fluorescein angiography is essential in the assessment of diabetic retinopathy, both in diagnosis and in the planning of treatment. The angiogram reveals the full extent of abnormalities of the retinal capillary bed, which are often found to be much more widespread and severe than the clinical appearances on ophthalmoscopy suggest (Plate VII). The extent of capillary non-perfusion can be demonstrated, an impossibility with either the ophthalmoscope or colour photographs, and the extent and type of maculopathy can be accurately assessed.

CLINICAL COURSE

The earliest features of diabetic retinopathy are increased retinal capillary permeability (i.e. break-down of the blood-retinal barrier) as demonstrated and measured by vitreous fluorophotometry, and capillary and venous dilatation. Both these manifestations can be reversed by strict metabolic control of the diabetes, at least in younger patients.

Simple Background Retinopathy (*Plate VII*)

The development of clinically apparent retinopathy implies the development of microaneurysms, dot and blot haemorrhages, and hard exudates.

Microaneurysms are found particularly at the posterior pole, and fluorescein angiography regularly reveals them to be much more numerous and widespread than is suspected clinically. When microaneurysms or damaged capillaries leak blood, dot and blot haemorrhages result, the former being deep in the retina and the latter in the superficial nerve fibre layer. Hard exudates result from leakage of lipid plasma constituents from abnormally permeable small vessels. They may remain small, scattered and discrete, or coalesce to form larger exudates which often occur as incomplete or complete rings around an area of capillary damage (circinate retinopathy).

Areas of retinal capillary occlusion are the most significant lesions of diabetic retinopathy, being the precursors to most of the serious progressive features of the condition. They are mainly found in the posterior fundus, including the macula, but wide-angle fluorescein angiographic photographs show that widespread capillary ischaemia is a common occurrence in the mid-peripheral retina, and that the extent of the non-perfusion parallels the severity of the retinopathy.

In the posterior fundus, where the nerve fibre layer is relatively thick, swelling and loss of transparency in the nerve fibres overlying areas of capillary non-perfusion results in the appearance of soft exudates or cottonwool spots. In the retinal mid-periphery where the nerve fibre layer is thinner, soft exudates are not usually seen, even when capillary ischaemia is extensive.

Background Retinopathy with Maculopathy (*Plates VIII–X*)

Maculopathy should be suspected whenever a patient with background retinopathy suffers a drop in visual acuity without other obvious cause such as cataract. Sometimes it is apparent as retinal oedema and concentration of the background lesions in the macular area, but in others it is not clinically obvious. In an elderly patient with early lens opacities, maculopathy may be missed if the significance of a drop in visual acuity is not recognized, and a fluorescein angiogram not obtained.

It is helpful to subdivide maculopathy into three types, which differ in their effect on vision and their progress (Whitelocke et al., 1979):

1. *Exudative,* or *focal (Plates VIII and IX)* : Here the predominant lesion is the leaking microaneurysm or damaged capillary. Groups of these lesions tend to occur focally at the macula, and exudate may form circles or parts of circles, with dot and blot haemorrhages in the centre. Fluorescein angiography shows the focal nature of the lesions, with late leakage of dye occurring at the areas of capillary damage, but adequate perfusion. When the fovea is not encroached upon, vision is initially good, and well preserved with time.

2. *Oedematous,* or *cystoid (Plate X)*: The macula can look surprisingly normal on ophthalmoscopy, but the fluorescein angiogram shows marked and generalized late leakage from the capillaries around the macula. The late frames of the angiogram show the characteristic petaloid pattern of cystoid macular oedema. Vision is much affected from the first, and visual prognosis is poor.

3. *Ischaemic:* Here again the macular oedema tends to be extensive and often cystoid in type. There are few exudates, but microaneurysms and haemorrhages. Fluorescein angiography shows evidence of capillary ischaemia extending to, and even across, the fovea. At the time of presentation vision is variably affected, but worsens in many cases, with the development of new vessels.

Preproliferative and Proliferative Retinopathy

These are uncommon over the age of 70, but occur more frequently in men than women, perhaps because of the effects of cigarette smoking (Aiello et al., 1983). With the progress of retinal ischaemia, the angiogram shows areas which do not fill with fluorescein and, around these, apparent attempts to revascularize the retina. Intraretinal microvascular abnormalities (IRMA) may be evident, and soft exudates may mark the ischaemic areas. Nerve fibre layer haemorrhages, of typical flame shape, also tend to increase with retinal ischaemia, and are often close to soft exudates. These occur in normotensive patients as well as those in whom hypertension is aggravating a purely diabetic retinopathy.

Background changes, plus IRMA and beading of the veins, together with perhaps soft exudates and extensive flame-shaped haemorrhages, represent a stage of background retinopathy which may be called 'preproliferative' because these frequently herald the appearance of frank neovascularization. It has been estimated that eyes with the features of preproliferative retinopathy have a 50 per cent chance of developing neovascularization in 1 year, untreated, and a 15 per cent chance of severe visual loss in 5 years (Diabetic Retinopathy Study Research Group, 1978, 1981).

Neovascularization at the disc or elsewhere in the retina with or without fibrous proliferation, and vitreous haemorrhage, are the hallmarks of the proliferative stage. If the retinal ischaemia is widespread enough, there may be neovascularization of the disc, and visual prognosis is then much worse.

As the neovascular membrane grows on the surface of the retina ('flat new vessels'), with or without accompanying fibroglial tissue proliferation, adhesion to the posterior hyaloid membrane tends to occur. Thus when the posterior vitreous face detaches forwards, the neovascular tissue is pulled with it ('forward new vessels') into the vitreous cavity. There is then a high risk of sight-threatening complications, in particular vitreous haemorrhage and retinal detachment.

TREATMENT

When diabetic retinopathy is diagnosed, especially when it is symptomatic, the doctor's natural reflex is to attempt to improve control of diabetes, in the hope that this will retard progression. There is, however, little evidence that at this stage improved control makes a critical difference to the prognosis of the condition in the elderly (Caird et al., 1969, *but see* Pirart, 1977). Enthusiasm for good control must always be tempered by the thought that the treatment must never be worse than the disease. Therapeutic effort should be concentrated on the early years of diabetes (*see above*), and in establishing and maintaining proper patterns of diet, therapy, and control of treatment. Nor must it be forgotten that diabetes in the elderly need not of itself be a great disability, and that the many and varied non-diabetic troubles of the elderly may greatly exceed diabetes as causes of problems for the patient. In elderly diabetics, the commonest sight-threatening complication is maculopathy, and factors which might favour its occurrence might be: greater and more erratic fluctuations of blood glucose levels in elderly diabetic patients, the proneness of elderly patients to be careless of their diabetic control, and the greater tendency of elderly people to have macular pathology of degenerative type.

Drug Treatment

A variety of drugs has been proposed for treatment of diabetic retinopathy, but because the natural course of the disease is so variable, and basic mechanisms underlying its development and progress still unknown, it is extremely difficult to assess the efficacy of drug treatment. Clofibrate has been shown in controlled studies to cause clearing of hard exudates in patients with exudative retinopathy, but the vascular lesions are unaffected and visual loss not reversed (Cullen et al., 1964). Recent studies of clofibrate and heart disease have suggested other potentially harmful effects.

Drugs which inhibit platelet aggregation, such as aspirin, have been proposed as treatment agents, because increased sensitivity of platelets to aggregation has been demonstrated in diabetics, and microvascular occlusive events may play a part in the aetiology of the retinopathy. Long-term controlled trials involving the use of aspirin are currently under way in the USA.

Photocoagulation

Photocoagulation is a destructive form of treatment, and why it is effective treatment is not yet understood. Photocoagulation with the intense white light of the xenon-arc was introduced for treatment of retinopathy by Meyer-Schwickerath in 1959, and the argon laser by L'Esperance in 1968. The latter employs a coherent blue and green beam which is absorbed by haemoglobin as well as by the retinal pigment epithelium. More recently a krypton laser has been introduced, which may prove effective while free of some of the argon laser's drawbacks.

Xenon-arc photocoagulation requires retrobulbar anaesthesia, but the argon laser needs only topical analgesia and a contact lens; it is relatively painless provided that the duration of the flash is kept short. With the argon laser the coagulation marks are smaller, less deep and gentler than with the xenon-arc, and can be applied with great precision both in regard to size of burn and position.

The main complications of treatment are slight constriction of the visual field, of which few patients seem aware, poor night vision, and an occasional drop in visual acuity due to macular oedema. Xenon-arc photocoagulation is more likely to produce these adverse effects than the argon laser.

Background Retinopathy

It is debatable whether photocoagulation has a place at this stage. Where fluorescein angiography shows an area of capillary non-perfusion, focal treatment may favourably influence the course of the condition. But more extensive photocoagulation of the whole retina is not justified, because the treatment itself carries a slight risk of damage to vision.

Maculopathy

Both xenon-arc and laser photocoagulation have been and are extensively used in this situation, and it is generally agreed that treatment confers a modest degree of protection to vision. It is important, before planning and starting treatment, to diagnose the predominant type of maculopathy.

　　1. *Exudative*, or *focal*:
　　　　The treatment is photocoagulation of the focal areas of micro-aneurysm formation with fluorescein leakage, including the

centres of the rings of exudate. Results of treatment in this form of maculopathy are good.

2. *Oedematous,* or *cystoid:*

Treatment consists of a grid of laser burns of low intensity, 50–100 μm in size, across the macular area, avoiding the papillo-macular bundle and within half the disc diameter of the fovea. Provided that treatment is instituted before the visual acuity has dropped greatly, the results are moderately encouraging. Panretinal photocoagulation is not indicated unless the angiogram shows a considerable amount of retinal ischaemia in the retinal mid-periphery.

3. *Ischaemia:*

Treatment of this type of maculopathy is difficult. Once again a grid of photocoagulation is used, as described above, and areas of ischaemia and of focal leakage are treated directly where possible.

The British Multicentre Study Group (1975) and Townsend et al. (1980) used the xenon-arc, and treatment was diffuse, to all visible lesions, plus either to the area temporal to the macula, or to the centre of rings of hard exudates where their position made this possible. The mean age of the 99 patients was only 58 years, and follow-up was 2–5 years. Visual acuity was maintained in the treated eyes, but deteriorated in the untreated eyes, reaching 2 lines of difference on the Snellen chart after 4 years. The best results were obtained in those with initially good vision, and no beneficial effect was found in patients whose initial visual acuity was less than 6/36.

A prospective randomized study using argon laser photocoagulation in 39 patients, with a 2-year follow-up, has been reported by Bankenship (1979). The treatment consisted of focal coagulation using 100 μm burns of areas showing fluorescein leakage, plus a grid pattern of 100 μm burns over the macula, sparing the papillomacular bundle and an area 0·5 disc diameter from the centre of the fovea. There was a tendency towards absorption of oedema and exudates in treated eyes, in contrast to untreated eyes, and visually the treated eyes did better. The results, while not statistically significant in the numbers studied, strongly suggested a trend towards treatment benefit, and eyes with initially good vision did best.

While treatment confers a degree of protection, this is not as dramatic as in proliferative retinopathy. The treatment itself, at the macula, must cause some damage, and other factors such as the 'premature ageing' which takes place in the diabetic patient's vasculature, and 'normal' senile macular degeneration probably play their part.

Table 10.1 shows results of the main published studies. The longest follow-up period has been 5 years, by Townsend et al. (1980). Their results showed that treated eyes maintained visual acuities during this

Table 10.1 Results of Photocoagulation for Diabetic Retinopathy

Author	Xenon-arc or argon laser	No. of patients	Pre-treatment visual acuity	Max. Follow-up (yrs)	Maintained or improved visual acuity (%)	
					Treated	Untreated
Controlled Randomised Studies						
1	Xenon (some laser)	63	6/12 or less	3	93	37
2 and 3	Xenon	99	6/6 to 6/24	5	69	37
4	Argon	39	6/12 to 6/36	2	77	57
Other Studies						
5	Xenon	20	6/6 to HM	2	80	—
6	Xenon	112	6/6 to <6/60	4	92	61
7	Argon	40	6/6 to 6/60	2	100 (focal) 90 (cystoid) 68 (ischaemic)	—
8	Argon	105	6/6 to CF	3	80	—

Key: 1: Patz et al. (1973).
2: British Multicentre Study (1975).
3: Townsend et al. (1980).
4: Bankenship (1979).
5: Spalter (1971) (only circinate maculopathy included).
6: Rubenstein and Myska (1974).
7: Whitelocke et al. (1979) (definitions of maculopathy as in text).
8: Reeser et al. (9181) (only circinate maculopathy included).

time, whereas untreated eyes, which had not shown much difference at the end of 2–3 years, thereafter deteriorated more markedly. This suggests that the results of treatment may be better the longer the follow-up.

Preproliferative Retinopathy

The optimum time for panretinal photocoagulation treatment in diabetic retinopathy has not yet been shown. Treatment carries its own risk of adverse effects, arguing for postponement of photocoagulation for as long as possible. On the other hand, the eye with preproliferative retinopathy has a high risk of developing new vessels, and it may require more extensive photocoagulation to cause established new vessels to regress than it does to prevent their appearance. These considerations argue for early treatment.

It is to be hoped that a multicentre trial in the USA, which eventually will involve 4,000 patients and over 20 centres (The Early Treatment of Diabetic Retinopathy Study), will provide an answer.

Proliferative Retinopathy

Panretinal photocoagulation is an effective treatment where new vessels are present on the optic disc. It may be that with the xenon-arc fewer sessions of treatment are needed, and quicker regression of new vessels obtained, and a few patients prefer it to the laser. However, the latter has the advantages of ease of application and lack of side effects, and it is the method of choice in most clinics.

Proliferative retinopathy with new vessels elsewhere than on the optic disc is more slowly progressive, and convincing benefits from photocoagulation have not so far been demonstrated.

SUMMARY

Diabetic retinopathy is now treatable, and we can prevent blindness in a large proportion of elderly patients. In addition to good control, now shown convincingly to be effective in decreasing the occurrence and severity of the retinopathy, patients who need photocoagulation must be recognized in good time and treated thoroughly. This treatment is time-consuming, tiring for patient and doctor, and tedious if it were not so rewarding in terms of prevention of visual deterioration.

REFERENCES

Aiello L. M., Rand L. I., Briones J. C. et al. (1983) In: Little H. L., Patz A., Jack R. L. and Forsham P. H. (eds) *Diabetic Retinopathy.* New York, Thieme-Stratton, p. 21.
Bankenship G. W. (1979) *Ophthalmology (Rochester)* **86,** 69.
British Multicentre Study Group (1975) *Lancet* **2,** 1110.
Burditt A. F., Caird F. I. and Draper G. J. (1968) *Q.J. Med. N.S.* **37,** 303.

Caird F. I. (1965) *Experta Med. Int. Congr. Ser.* **84**, 465.

Caird F. I. (1982) In: Evans J. G. and Caird F. I. *Advanced Geriatric Medicine* **2**, London, Pitman Medical, p. 3.

Caird F. I., Pirie A. and Ramsell T. G. (1969) *Diabetes and the Eye.* Oxford, Blackwell.

Committee on Blindness (1970) London, British Diabetic Association.

Constam G. R. (1965) *Helv. Med. Acta* **32**, 287.

Cullen J. F., Ireland J. T. and Oliver M. F. (1964) *Trans. Ophthalmol. Soc. UK.* **84**, 281.

Diabetic Retinopathy Study Research Group (1978) *Ophthalmol. (Rochester)* **85**, 82.

Diabetic Retinopathy Study Research Group (1981) *Ophthalmol. (Rochester)* **88**, 583.

Leslie R. D. G., Barnett A. H. and Pyke D. A. (1979) *Lancet* **1**, 997.

Patz A., Schatz H., Berkow J. W. et al. (1973) *Trans. Am. Acad. Ophthalmol. Otolaryngol.* **77**, 34.

Pirart J. (1977) *Diabete Metab.* **3**, 97, 173 and 245.

Reeser F., Fleishman J., Williams J. A. et al. (1981) *Am. J. Ophthalmol.* **92**, 762.

Rubinstein R. and Myska V. (1974) *Br. J. Ophthalmol.* **58**, 77.

Soler N. G., Fitzgerald M. G., Malins J. M. et al. (1969) *Br. Med. J.* **3**, 567.

Spalter H. F. (1971) *Am. J. Ophthalmol.* **71**, 242.

Townsend C., Bailey J. and Kohner E. (1980) *Br. J. Ophthalmol.* **64**, 385.

Whitelocke R. A. F., Kearns M., Blach R. K. et al. (1979) *Trans. Ophthalmol. Soc. UK* **84**, 281.

11. RETINAL VASCULAR DISEASE
T. Barrie

This chapter discusses aspects of retinal vascular disease which occur commonly in the elderly. In addition, retinal vascular diseases which occur across the age range are discussed with particular reference to those which may differ in the elderly. There is often little difference between the management of these conditions in different age groups, but where appropriate these differences are mentioned.

RETINAL ARTERIAL OCCLUSIONS

In the elderly, branch or central retinal arterial occlusions may occur consequent upon atherosclerotic disease of the carotid circulation or much less commonly, as a result of giant cell arteritis affecting more distal areas of the circulation. Whilst the obvious case of giant cell arteritis is unlikely to be missed, particularly if the typical symptoms of polymyalgia rheumatica and temporal arteritis are present, it is mandatory to exclude this diagnosis since the second eye may be affected by a retinal arterial occlusion within 24–48 hours of the first eye in the absence of appropriate treatment. The sudden onset of total blindness in an elderly person is completely devastating, and will often have the most far reaching consequences upon that patient's ability to live independently (*see* Chapter 15). With this background in mind, it is appropriate to consider the clinical presentation of giant cell arteritis, quite apart from its ophthalmic involvement. The original description by Hutchinson (1889) of temporal arteritis describes exquisitely tender red streaks crossing the scalp, but often this condition is not seen at such an advanced stage and the symptoms of temporal arteritis are simply of a pulsatile headache typically superficial in origin and associated with tenderness of the skin of the scalp in the region of the temporal arteries, which should themselves be palpable. Whether or not they are pulsatile will depend on whether or not the vessel is occluded.

Polymyalgia rheumatica usually presents with symptoms of pain and stiffness affecting the limbs and shoulder girdle muscles, typically worse of waking. A further important feature not given sufficient emphasis is that there is often a complaint of a very nondescript general malaise over the preceding few months, and the comments of the spouse may be particularly helpful in describing the patient as having been 'just not himself', feeling generally lethargic and listless, often accompanied by a change of mood, with the patient becoming increasingly ill-tempered. In view of the importance of identifying giant cell arteritis as a cause of retinal arterial occlusion, it is important to elicit such symptoms, which may not be volunteered at the time of presentation with acute visual loss.

Clinical Appearance of Retinal Arterial Occlusion

Typically an acute obstruction of the central retinal artery or a branch retinal artery manifests itself as a sudden loss or decrease of vision in one eye. However, it is not uncommon in elderly patients for such loss not to be noted for some time; it may indeed only be found as a result of closing the good eye or in the course of an examination by an optician. In the acute stage, the clinical signs should be quite obvious with a distinctive white appearance to the affected area of the retina, caused by intracellular oedema as a result of reduced perfusion (*Plate XI* 1). This retinal oedema obscures the underlying choroid, giving rise to the white appearance, but since the retina is thinnest at the fovea, the underlying choroidal vasculature remains more obvious here, so giving rise to the so-called 'cherry red spot' (*Plate XI* 2). This is often not nearly as obvious as is normally suggested in standard textbooks. Where the occlusion has occurred as a result of cholesterol emboli dislodged from atheromatous plaques, fragments of these emboli may be seen through the retinal arterioles as discreet refractile bodies visible at the bifurcation of the vessels where the diameter becomes reduced, so trapping the emboli prior to their fragmentation into smaller emboli. Where the presentation is not so acute, the retinal oedema may be far from obvious. In the late stages, the retina itself may look entirely normal, but the retinal arteries are abnormally thin and attenuated, with eventual secondary pallor of the optic disc, consequent upon degeneration of the nerve fibre layer of the retina.

Treatment

Once the retinal arterial occlusion has occurred, treatment aimed at re-establishing flow along the occluded vessel is of very limited effect. Moreover, the assessment of treatment is difficult, since spontaneous improvement may occur. Whilst the full spectrum of treatment as described is far from appropriate for every patient, the fitter the patient and the more recent the occlusion, the more aggressive should the treatment be. In particular, when the occlusion appears to have occurred within a few hours, functional recovery following re-establishment of flow might be expected to occur if the intra-ocular pressure can be reduced rapidly. If the plasma viscosity can be reduced, this may further encourage re-establishment of retinal blood flow.

It is traditional to administer acetazolamide (Diamox) to lower the intra-ocular pressure, but it may be more effective to attempt to dislodge emboli by sudden lowering of the intra-ocular pressure by surgical removal of some of the aqueous humour. This can be done by paracentesis at the slit-lamp, only topical local anaesthesia being required. Rebound rise in intra-ocular pressure following paracentesis can be controlled with acetazolamide. Should the patient be seen in circumstances where paracentesis is not possible, a reduction in intra-ocular pressure may be achieved by vigorous massage to the eye.

Infusions of low molecular weight dextrans have been tried in an effort to lower the plasma viscosity. It is now argued that the net effect of these agents on plasma viscosity may be minimal. It might be more appropriate to give an osmotic diuretic such as mannitol, either orally or intravenously, since this will achieve decreased plasma viscosity as a result of increasing the intravascular volume, and also maintain an adequate perfusion pressure. In elderly patients, such a régime should not be embarked upon if it is felt that this could precipitate cardiac failure.

Embolic retinal arterial occlusion is a manifestation of carotid atherosclerosis. The carotid circulation should be assessed in more detail since retinal arterial occlusions are caused by the same mechanism as transient ischaemic attacks, and it should be realized that the prognosis for a subsequent cerebrovascular accident is similar. In the elderly, it is most unlikely that surgery such as carotid endarterectomy would be considered, and there is therefore no question of performing carotid angiography. Doppler ultrasound scanning of the carotids can be helpful in assessing the carotid situation in a totally non-invasive manner (Dodson et al., 1982). In the elderly the only treatment offered may be low-dose aspirin in order to reduce platelet adhesiveness and so reduce the build-up of clot on the atheromatous plaques in the carotid arteries.

In the treatment of a retinal arterial occlusion caused by giant cell arteritis it is essential that systemic steroids be given in adequate dosage as soon as possible. The rationale for giving steroids is not to improve the function of the affected eye, but to prevent an occlusion in the fellow eye. An accepted treatment is 200 mg hydrocortisone intravenously, and 80–120 mg prednisolone per day orally. Difficulties may arise where there is only a suspicion that giant cell arteritis may be the cause; in these circumstances, it should be remembered that there is often a delay of a few days in the erythrocyte sedimentation rate (ESR) rising, and a normal ESR should therefore not refute a clinical diagnosis of giant cell arteritis as a cause of a retinal arterial occlusion. Once the acute stage has been brought under control, it is particularly important in elderly patients to reduce the dose of systemic steroids as rapidly as possible. In giant cell arteritis, both the ESR and the patient's general symptoms (headache from temporal arteritis or the more general symptoms of polymyalgia rheumatica) indicate whether dosage is adequate. It is usually possible for the dose of prednisolone to be reduced to around 20 mg within two weeks; it is often much more difficult to reduce the dose further, attempts being thwarted by the rise in ESR together with the return of symptoms. The patient may often require up to 10 mg prednisolone daily for up to two years before the disease burns itself out. Should the disease be inadequately treated, then there is a significant risk that further vascular occlusions in either the ophthalmic or cerebral arteries may occur.

RETINAL VENOUS OCCLUSION

Like venous occlusions elsewhere in the body these may be predisposed to by increased viscosity of the blood disease, affecting the vessel wall, or pressure from without giving rise to narrowing or obliteration of the vein lumen. In the elderly, the most common predisposing factors are from without but increased plasma viscosity may also be of considerable relevance. Clinically, retinal venous occlusions can be classified into *central*, where the veins occlude within or behind the cribiform plate; *hemisphere*, when the vein is occluded at the optic disc after dividing into an upper and lower trunk, but before dividing into quadrants; or *branch*, affecting one of the quadrants or its tributaries.

Central Retinal Vein Occlusion

This presents as a sudden loss of vision in one eye, but (as mentioned regarding arterial occlusions), an elderly person may be slower to notice this. The clinical appearance is typically of extensive retinal haemorrhages, which are mainly in the inner retina, and therefore flame-shaped (*Plate XII* 1). There are, however, haemorrhages in the deeper retina which are round. The macular retina is likely to be oedematous and there may also be cottonwool spots (soft exudates). The retinal veins appear dilated and tortuous, and often the disc itself may be swollen. Vision will be significantly reduced in the acute stage but, depending on a variety of factors, it may eventually recover almost completely; the eye may become both painful and blind from glaucoma due to neovascularization of the iris (rubeosis). One of the main factors which influences the final visual outcome is the extent of collateral circulation. This develops more readily if the obstruction is gradual rather than complete and sudden. Fluorescein angiography is helpful in assessing the prognosis. Adverse factors are extensive leakage from dilated capillaries, giving rise to macular oedema and, more importantly, large areas of capillary non-perfusion. The latter suggests that visual outcome will be poor, and that there will be a high chance of rubeotic glaucoma, typically within two or three months or so of the occlusion. Where capillary closure is extensive, multiple cottonwool spots are readily visible; these represent impaired axoplasmic flow consequent upon significant retinal ischaemia (McLeod et al., 1977).

In hemisphere vein occlusion, the fundal changes are essentially similar, but localized only to the half of the retina drained by the occluded veins (*Plate XII* 2). The same comments regarding prognostic features in central retinal vein occlusion also apply here. In cases of chronic simple glaucoma with significant cupping of the optic discs, this type of venous occlusion may occur where the veins bend acutely to dip into the pathologically deep cup of the optic disc.

In a branch retinal vein occlusion, the appearances are of haemorrhages together with hard exudates localized to the quadrant drained by the affected vein. On fundoscopy it should be possible to identify the site of occlusion since this is almost invariably where the vein is 'nipped' by the overlying artery (*Plate XIII*). Where a temporal vein is involved, then the macula (and consequently central vision) will be affected, but where a nasal vein is occluded then only a temporal field defect will be noted, the visual acuity remaining normal. The prognostic features for visual outcome are very much the same as for hemisphere and central vein occlusions.

Treatment

Where there is significant capillary closure on the fluorescein angiogram in any vein occlusion, a vasoformative factor is thought to be elaborated by the underperfused retina. It is this presumed vasoformative factor which is responsible for the development of neovascular complications, such as disc and peripheral new vessels and iris vessels (rubeosis iridis) which may grow across the drainage angle and obliterate it giving rise to rubeotic glaucoma. Where capillary closure is identified at a sufficiently early stage, then scattered photocoagulation burns to the underperfused areas of the retina should be given in a manner similar to diabetes, the intention being to induce regression of the retinal and iris new vessels before irreversible complications ensue. Such treatment may be performed as an out-patient with only topical anaesthesia, and as such is eminently suitable for the elderly patient, the only proviso being that lens opacities are more likely to contribute to difficulties of treatment.

SYSTEMIC DISEASE

Where an elderly person has lost the sight in one eye the physician must try to identify any treatable predisposing factor in order to prevent a further occlusion in the other eye. Systemic hypertension has been shown to be the most common treatable predisposing factor in retinal vascular occlusion. However, in the elderly, AV nipping need not be a sign of systemic hypertension but rather a manifestation of arteriosclerosis of the retinal arterioles. Systemic hypertension should be treated as appropriate, bearing in mind the problems associated with the side effects of hypotensive drugs in the elderly.

A significant increase in plasma lipids has been found in patients with branch and central vein occlusions when compared to age-matched controls (Ring et al., 1976), but our own impression is that in the elderly this is uncommon, but should be looked for, since it is eminently treatable.

Increased plasma viscosity has been also recognized in particular in association with retinal vein occlusion, and especially those associated with significant capillary closure (Trope et al., 1983). The increased haematocrit is mostly the result of polycythaemia secondary to chronic obstructive airways disease, and attempts to lower the plasma viscosity by venesection are likely to be unsuccessful; where another cause of increased plasma viscosity is identified, it is worth while to try appropriate means of reducing it. Quite apart from a raised haematocrit, blood viscosity has been shown to be raised in retinal vein occlusions even when corrected to a standard haematocrit; the main cause appears to be a raised plasma fibrinogen, but it is arguable whether this is a relevant predisposing factor. In addition, plasma levels of antithrombin-III and Factor VIII are lower; it is therefore important to look for these, since they must indicate an increased risk to the other eye.

In summary, retinal venous occlusion is a common cause of visual deterioration in the elderly. It is important to assess and treat this condition actively, since ophthalmic treatment with photocoagulation may retain vision which would otherwise be lost from complications such as retinal and iris neovascularization. The importance of identifying and treating any general predisposing factors lies in reducing the chances of a similar occlusion affecting the other eye.

Hypertension

Hypertension is hard to define in the elderly. Its effect on the retinal vasculature is also quite different from that of hypertension in young to middle-aged patients.

The standard classification of hypertensive retinopathy has been for many years that described by Keith and Wagener, as follows:

Grade I: attenuation of retinal arteries
Grade II: similar but more marked changes than Grade I with nipping of the retinal veins where they are crossed by arteries
Grade III: there is in addition retinal oedema, linear haemorrhages, and cottonwool spots
Grade IV: as for Grade III, but with papilloedema

Whilst this is a helpful classification, particularly with regards to prognosis for life, it has its limits, and is really only valid for patients in whom there is no significant degree of arteriosclerosis, prior to the blood pressure becoming raised. This classification is not helpful when considering hypertensive retinal vascular changes in the elderly, where there has usually been a parallel development of arteriosclerosis and hypertension, with the hypertensive changes superimposed on a background of arteriosclerosis of the retinal vessels. The changes in the retinal vasculature consequent upon arteriosclerosis with a normal blood pressure are thinning and straightening of the retinal arterioles which may be a little irregular. There may in addition be quite obvious AV nipping. This would fall into Grade II hypertensive retinopathy by Keith and Wagener's classification, but in a normotensive elderly patient such an appearance can occur simply as a result of retinal arteriosclerosis.

When hypertension occurs in the elderly the retinal arterioles may become more irregular; the presumed explanation is that segments of the muscular wall of the arteriole have been replaced by fibrous tissue and are unable to contract, and this gives rise to the irregular calibre. AV nipping is likely to be much more obvious, and there may be noticeable dilatation of the vein on the distal side of the crossing. With hypertension of longer duration and greater severity in the elderly, the degree of retinal arteriosclerosis is such that most of the muscle in the retinal arterioles has changed to fibrous tissue, and the vessels have lost their contractile ability. They therefore cannot respond to the high intraluminal pressure by hypertrophy of the muscle wall, and a stage of decompensation arises, allowing egress of constituents of plasma into the extravascular tissues. This is manifest clinically by the appearance of hard exudates; these represent lipid-laden macrophages which have engulfed debris and are attempting to remove it from the retina. This is a manifestation of arteriosclerosis rather than hypertension *per se*. Hard exudates may be scattered, or in the pattern of a macular star. When the hypertension is more severe, cottonwool spots appear, representing impaired axoplasmic flow along the nerve fibre layer of the retina. It is uncommon for elderly patients to develop the grossest hypertensive retinopathy, but when it does occur the optic disc may be swollen.

The treatment of hypertensive retinopathy is treatment of the hypertension. In younger patients there is a dramatic and rapid improvement in the retinopathy following reduction of the blood pressure to normal levels. But in the elderly this improvement is likely to be much slower and less striking, since the retinopathy is contributed to quite significantly by arteriosclerosis, and is unaffected by subsequent control of the blood pressure. Nevertheless, the decreased intraluminal pressure would be expected to induce a reduction in the number of haemorrhages, hard exudates, and cottonwool spots, but not perhaps as rapidly as would be expected in a younger patient with a less arteriosclerotic retinal vascular tree.

REFERENCES

Dodson P. M., Galton D. J., Hamilton A. M. et al. (1982) *Br. J. Opthalmol.* **66,** 161.

Hutchison J. (1889) *Arch. Surg.* **1,** 323.

McLeod D., Marshall J., Kohner E. M. et al. (1977) *Br. J. Ophthalmol.* **61,** 177.

Ring C. P., Pearson T. C., Saunders M. D. et al. (1976) *Br. J. Ophthalmol.* **60,** 397.

Trope G. E., Lowe G. D. O., Shafour I. M. et al. (1983) *Trans. Ophthalmol. Soc. UK.* **103,** 108.

12. DISPLACEMENTS OF THE RETINA
Hector B. Chawla

INTRODUCTION

Talk of the developed retina can frighten potential observers, and its embryology can be daunting. However, it is necessary to retain a few facts about its origin. It makes its appearance in the embryo as a balloon arising from the ectoderm of the forebrain. The anterior portion of this balloon, growing more slowly than the posterior, dimples and continues to dimple, finally sinking into the cavity to form two layers. The inner layer becomes the neuro-retina, and the outer the pigment retina, which provides protection against excess light, mottles the choroidal red and masks the scleral white. Between them lies a natural line of cleavage, The anterior fold marks the union of the two layers in the formed retina, becoming the ora serrata, which lies deep to a line connecting the insertions of the four rectus muscles.

The neuro-retina, as part of the brain, is not without its complexities, but the details need not concern us. The essentials can be reduced to light receptors lying adjacent to the pigment retina, connecting through a series of cell stations, and finally ending as nerve fibres next to the vitreous. These fibres arrive from all areas of the retina, and funnel out of the eye as the optic nerve at the optic disc.

When we speak of the retina, we tend to mean one, the neuro-retina, but anatomically there are two, with a natural line of cleavage between them. When any influence separates the inner from the outer, we have a displacement (detachment) of the retina.

CAUSES OF DETACHMENT

The retina may be displaced in three basic ways and, for the sake of completeness, a fourth form has been included, which looks like a displacement but is not.

1. Fluid may collect in the space of cleavage. This occurs most frequently when a break in the neuro-retina allows liquid vitreous to fill the potential space. Fluid may collect in the space for other reasons, but the appearances will be the same.

119

2. Traction may pull the neuro-retina into the vitreous cavity, as is commonly seen in proliferative diabetic retinopathy.
3. Any space-occupying lesion, meeting less resistance to inward than to outward spread, will raise the neuro-retina. Since it will always raise the pigment retina as well, the term 'solid retinal detachment' is not wholly accurate, but that is the name that is most popular (*Plate XIV* 1).
4. An unnatural line of cleavage may sometimes develop within the neuro-retina. This does not develop without filling with fluid, and producing cyst formation, which can give the impression of a retinal detachment.

SYMPTOMS

A detaching retina produces a defect in the visual field, which the patient may not notice until the macula is detached as well, and then the complaint will be of sudden loss of central vision. Should the detachment be sudden, the field defect must be noticed by the patient, but will not normally take precedence over the more startling features which come before it.

The vitreous may tug on the retina intermittently, resulting in the impression of recurrent and persistent flashing lights. Should blood, pigment, or retinal debris be released into the vitreous as the result of a retinal break, the patient will complain of a sudden shower of 'floaters'. Many people notice floaters, but the distinctive feature of importance is how long they have been present, their suddenness of origin, and their companions. Floaters noticed casually over five years may be intrinsically little different from floaters noticed within the past five minutes. But the dramatic onset, the flashing lights, and finally the field defect, must make clear to patient and doctor which floaters are to be taken seriously.

SIGNS

The healthy fundal reflex is caused by the choroid glowing red through the pigment retina, the latter varying in darkness according to its thickness, and also to race. Before them all lies the neuro-retina, transparent when flat, but grey when detached, rippling if mobile, and crossed by curving dark blood vessels in focus in general only with the plus lens of the ophthalmoscope (*Plate XIV* 2). The binocular indirect ophthalmoscope allows a panoramic view of the entire retina, beyond the equator and out to the ora serrata, where most of the breaks are to be found. All eyes suspected of detachment must be examined with this instrument.

SIMPLE RETINAL DETACHMENT

Degenerate vitreous seeps through a break in the neuro-retina into the natural space of cleavage. The neuro-retina is separated from its deep blood supply, and will eventually stop seeing altogether, unless the separation is overcome. The macula, requiring more blood than the rest of the neuro-retina, always declines somewhat in function, even after the briefest of separations.

Detachment is more common in myopes, because the myopic eye is large, the retina is thin, and perforations more likely. Aphakic eyes develop breaks behind the ora serrata, where the normally adherent vitreous is disturbed by the cataract extraction. Breaks also occur in other parts of the retina, such as the macula and the ora serrata as the result of injury. Neither is particularly common in the elderly.

Management: There is no alternative to surgery. If the problem is of recent onset, with the preservation of central vision, then the matter is obviously of some urgency, to preserve macular function at its highest level. The aim of surgery is to find the retinal break and seal it. Sealing is produced by inflammation, at the present time with a freezing pencil (cryopexy). The area of retina bearing the break has to be held against the underlying inflammation long enough to bind all the tissues together with a permanent watertight scar (*Plate XV* 1). In general the retinal tear will not remain in the correct position unless it is persuaded to do so, either by direction from within, or by indentation from without.

A break may be floated upwards against the 'glue' by an air bubble injected into the vitreal cavity. 24–36 hours suffice to float the break into position, but the air bubble may take several more days to absorb. If an air bubble is not possible, then all the layers of the eye may be pushed inwards to raise a 'buckle' connecting the 'glue' with the retinal break. This buckle is raised by stitching an explant of silicone rubber or Silastic sponge onto the outside of the sclera. Occasionally both methods may be necessary if there is any suggestion that the retina is going to pull off again. The essential principle is that the combined strength of the 'glue' and the buckle holding the retina flat should be greater than any traction force trying to pull it off again.

Surgery, if carried out by a retinal surgeon, should produce a functioning retina at the first attempt with little postoperative morbidity. Any ocular surgery results in inflammation which is not necessarily due to infection. It may produce an iritis, which may result in effusion of inflammatory fluid or the more chronic production of adhesions. The inflammatory effusion may silt up the drainage angle, resulting in acute secondary glaucoma. The more chronic problems may make the iris adhere to the lens and prevent the normal flow of aqueous fluid.

After operation, atropine drops are used to dilate the pupil. This prevents the iris from sticking to the lens in the constricted position;

corticosteroid drops reduce the tendency for it to stick in any position. Antibiotics, either local or systemic, are not prescribed as a routine. The pain of correctly performed surgery should not require more than simple analgesics after the patient has been discharged from hospital. An eye pad serves two functions. The first is to prevent light from dazzling the retina through the dilated pupil. The second is to mop up the excessive tears produced by surgical intervention. If the eye is not dazzled, and has stopped watering, then the pad may be discarded. In the past patients were confined to bed before and after operation. However, recent evidence suggests that nothing is to be gained, and especially in the elderly this immobility may be positively dangerous. In general recovery should be complete by 4 weeks after surgery.

RETINAL DETACHMENT DUE TO TRACTION

This most commonly complicates diabetic retinopathy, and indeed in the elderly may be the presenting feature of diabetes.

Management: As with simple detachment the aim is to close the break, but the contracting membranes in the vitreal cavity may continue to keep it open. In addition, a diabetic eye is already ischaemic, and does not tolerate surgery well. An attempt may therefore be made with a conventional operation, but because the presenting feature is traction, the retina may drag off again, if indeed it ever flattens (*Plate XV* 2).

In recent years improved microsurgical techniques have made it possible to enter the vitreal cavity itself, and on occasion to remove obscuring membranes, blood, and fibrous vitreous bands. A micro-probe which cuts and sucks can be inserted into the eye anterior to the rectus muscle insertions, where it cannot cut an unwanted hole in the retina. Simultaneously the eye is prevented from collapsing by a flow of normal saline through another hole ahead of the ora serrata, balancing the volume of vitreous and contents removed.

The diabetic eye in particular may bleed, and the bleeding points can be coagulated with underwater diathermy. Once the operation is complete and the retina flat and the bleeding points secure, then attention may be turned to the underlying retinopathy. A clear eye is necessary if this is to be carried out in the standard fashion with the laser, but in these eyes it may be technically easier to carry out the treatment from inside with a light coagulation probe, which can be fired directly at the retina.

SENILE MACULAR DEGENERATION

Degeneration of the macula, with its resultant destruction of central vision, is a common cause of visual disability in the elderly (*see* Chapter 9). The macula, as mentioned above, is vulnerable to the slightest variation in blood supply, and uses more blood per unit area than any other part of the retina. Indeed it is this very flow of blood that is sometimes blamed for mechanical disruption of the underlying layers in old age. 'Cracks' in Bruch's membrane between the pigment retina and the choroid develop and allow tissue fluid to pass into the potential space between, elevating the macula. In due course the fluid will be followed by new blood vessels and finally by blood. Occasionally this elevation of the macula retina detaches the retina much as it would detach if the macula were actually perforated. Such perforations are more common in high myopes and eyes that have sustained a blunt injury.

Management: A retinal detachment due to a macular hole must be treated like any other detachment, and the price paid for the restoration of the remaining field vision is the loss of whatever central vision remains. It is this threat to the remaining field that makes patients recognize just how important this segment of vision can be, whose existence they neither knew of nor understood.

If the retina itself is intact, but has elevated due to the leakage of fluid through the cracked barriers deep to the retina, then there is no threat to the field, but there is more than a threat to the centre. Occasionally it is possible to identify the exact spot where the normal tissue barriers have broken down, by fluorescein angiography. Leaking 'cracks' can be sealed by laser photocoagulation. If the defect lies across the macula central vision may be permanently lost. The further it is from the macula, the better the chance of visual recovery.

SCLERITIS*

Inflammation of the slera occurs more often than it is diagnosed. It follows the pattern of a granulomatous inflammation of collagen, often associated with rheumatoid arthritis and similar diseases. However, it has been known to develop in eyes where the sclera is the seat of some insult, not uncommonly surgical.

One of the characteristics of inflammation is the swelling due to an abnormal collection of fluid, and, given the normal anatomy of the retina, the normal space of cleavage is the only space that can fill easily with inflammatory fluid. If the inflammatory component is mild enough to escape notice, the subsequent retinal detachment can easily be misdiagnosed as simple, but one where the retinal break has proved elusive. The first step to diagnosis is to recognize that there may be no retinal break, and that scleritis is more common than was previously thought.

---

*For another view, *see* Chapter 5

The treatment is certainly not surgical. Certain cases may respond to non-steroidal anti-inflammatory agents, either in the short or the long term. It is only by noting the speed of response that one will determine which condition falls into which category.

The more severe varieties require a combination of immunosuppressive drugs and corticosteroids in relatively high doses. No matter what the age group, such regimes carry their problems and have to be monitored by those experienced in such matters.

Without treatment the eye can suffer irreparable damage from acute inflammation, from necrosis and the fibrous replacement of special tissue. The intra-ocular pressure can rise because of inflammatory disruption of the drainage mechanism, and may subsequently collapse as the same process destroys the ciliary body. The cornea can lose its clarity and the sclera its substance, turning from white to blue as the choroid becomes visible from the outside. If the lens remains clear, which it probably will not, the retina will be seen to have shrunk into a knotted fibrous sightless tangle.

Whatever is the ultimate combination of drugs chosen, it must be evident that the first step to avoid disaster is to recognize that the detachment is not amenable to surgery.

SPACE-OCCUPYING LESIONS

'Solid detachment' of the retina (*Plate XIV* 1) may occur when some space-occupying mechanism raises the choroid, the pigment retina, and the neuro-retina towards the vitreal cavity, either as a result of haemorrhage into the choroid, or of a tumour, primary or secondary. Causes of choroidal haemorrhage include hypertension (top of the list of possibilities), diabetes and bleeding disorders.

Of the tumours, malignant melanoma, although the most common in non-pigmented races, occurs in only about 1 in 40 000 of the population, and is almost invariably unilateral. As its progress is slow, symptoms are also slow, and may not be noticed until late in the disease. They usually relate to disturbance of retinal function. However, anterior tumours may invade the drainage angle, raising intra-ocular pressure with some rapidity and such pain that it may be mistaken for acute closed-angled glaucoma.

The real problem with melanoma is that by the time of its discovery it may already have spread, and the trauma of surgery may spread it even further. In the past the traditional approach was enucleation, but in recent years local excision of the melanoma, provided it is small enough, has become possible. The decision to operate must be justified, and perhaps the greatest justification is the preservation of vision in an only eye. However, given the finality of enucleation, there might be something to be said in favour of considering the preservation of vision in an eye.

If any doubt hangs over the diagnosis, a less definitive line of action is to photograph the offending mass and compare its appearance every six months with that in the first photograph. Should serial pictures demonstrate an increase in size, then removal of the tumour might be considered, and indeed should always be considered before removal of the eye itself. Such surgery is in its infancy, and perhaps not as successful now as it may be in the future, but it has already advanced enough to give the lie to its more cynical name of 'two-stage enucleation'.

Secondary tumours should not be forgotten, although they tend to be bilateral, but even more they tend to be rather rare. Common primary sources are breast and lung (*see* Chapter 2).

RETINOSCHISIS

This condition is not so much a displacement of the retina as an appearance of the same. The neuro-retina is not displaced, but is still in contact with the pigment retina. The neuro-retina splits, and fluid collects in the space left by the collapse of its middle layers. Thus a cyst is produced within the neuro-retina. The deep part remains in contact with the pigment retina and the choroid, while the inner leaf of the cyst masquerades as a retinal detachment.

But there are differences which can be seen with the ophthalmoscope —not least the smooth taut wall of the cyst, which is quite unlike the rippling contours of a detachment. There is the almost invariable absence of symptoms unless, as rarely happens, the condition spreads to involve the posterior pole. Retinoschisis is thus usually an incidental finding.

Management: This hinges on recognizing that the condition is not a retinal detachment, and that the only problems arise through ill-advised surgery. In those rare cases where it does spread far enough to cause symptoms, a barrage of light coagulation may halt its spreading edge. The rationale of this treatment assumes that the edge is in fact spreading.

FURTHER READING

Duke-Elder Sir Stewart and Dobree J. H. (eds.) (1967) Diseases of the retina. In: *Duke-Elder's System of Ophthalmology,* Vol. X, pp. 711–856. London, Kimpton.

Freeman H. M., Hirose T. and Schepens C. L. (1977) Vitreous surgery. In: *Advances in Fundus Diagnosis and Treatment.* New York: Appleton Century Crofts, pp. 279–304.

Schutz J. S. (1984) *Retinal Detachment Surgery: Strategy and Tactics.* London, Chapman & Hall Medical.

13. DISORDERS OF THE OPTIC NERVE
Swithin P. Meadows

Disorders of the optic nerve in the elderly differ from those in young and middle age largely in the pathology of the affecting agent. Giant-cell or temporal arteritis is almost confined to the elderly, and rarely occurs in patients under the age of 60 years. Arteriosclerotic involvement of the nerve is common in the middle-aged and elderly (as is diabetic retinopathy) and unusual in the young. Retrobulbar and optic neuritis are rare in the elderly, except perhaps tobacco amblyopia. Compression of the optic nerve by tumour or aneurysm may occur at almost any age.

Anatomy: The optic nerve is about 5 cm in length and extends from the globe posteriorly to the optic foramen (3 cm), transverses the optic canal to become intracranial and, finally, joins the optic chiasm on each side. The intra-orbital portion is slightly sinuous to allow free movement of the eyeball. In the orbit the nerve is surrounded by dura, arachnoid and pia, but the intracranial portion has only a pial covering. The subarachnoid space surrounding the intra-orbital portion of the nerve is continuous with the intracranial subarachnoid space via the optic canal, and contains a small amount of cerebrospinal fluid. This has some relevance to the development of papilloedema due to raised intracranial pressure, the latter being transmitted to the perineural sheath of the intra-orbital portion of the nerve. At the chiasm the medial or nasal fibres of each nerve, representing the temporal field of vision, decussate and finally join the contralateral optic tract, along with the lateral or temporal fibres from the other optic nerve, so that each optic tract contains fibres representing the homonymous visual fields of the opposite side. A brief description of the vascular relations of the optic nerve occurs later.

Diagnosis: The diagnosis of optic nerve disorder depends largely upon accurate and detailed clinical observation. Further investigations are often needed but cannot replace the initial clinical study. The history of visual failure, whether abrupt or gradual in onset, and the presence of other ophthalmic symptoms, such as visual hallucinations, temporary visual obscurations, diplopia, ocular pain or headache, is crucial. General medical and neurological examination may be of considerable assistance in diagnosis, including any history of angina, dyspnoea, disturbance of limbs (sensory or motor), or previous episodes of neurological dysfunction. A total history is of paramount importance.

Examination of the functions of the optic nerve may be summarized as follows:

1. Detailed ophthalmoscopic examination of the optic disc, retinal vessels, macula and periphery of the retina.
2. Corrected visual acuity in each eye (and colour vision).
3. Visual fields: an initial examination by confrontation tests, using a long-headed white hat pin, may produce evidence of a local defect in the visual field, such as a central scotoma, hemianopia or other field loss, to be confirmed later by more detailed examination on the perimeter or Bjerrum screen.

General medical examination, including that of the heart, peripheral arteries, blood pressure and urine, and a complete neurological examination are essential, as well as inspection for any evidence of dyspituitarism.

VASCULAR DISORDERS OF THE OPTIC NERVE

Anatomy: The ophthalmic artery arises from the internal carotid as the latter emerges from the cavernous sinus, and passes through the optic canal within the dural sheath of the optic nerve. It lies at first inferior and then lateral to the nerve, and in the orbit crosses above the nerve to reach the medial wall of the orbit.

The branches of ophthalmic importance are the central retinal artery and the posterior ciliary arteries (*Fig.* 13.1). The central retinal artery arises near the optic foramen below the optic nerve, then bends upwards to enter it, and finally forwards in the centre of the nerve to the lamina cribrosa which it pierces to enter the eye. After penetration of the nerve the central retinal artery is virtually an end artery to supply the retina. The posterior ciliary arteries arising from the ophthalmic artery divide into 10–20 small branches (short posterior ciliaries) which surround the optic nerve and pass forwards to pierce the eyeball around the optic nerve. These arteries form an arterial circle (circle of Zinn) which surrounds the optic nerve head inside the sclera, and supplies the papilla and anterior portion of the optic nerve. Two branches of the ophthalmic artery, the long posterior ciliaries, lie one on each side of the optic nerve, and pierce the sclera to supply the uveal tract.

The optic nerve and papilla are thus supplied by a network of small vessels, derived from the ophthalmic artery and its posterior ciliary and other branches, as distinct from the retina which is supplied by the central retinal artery. This is of some clinical significance in the production of ischaemic papillopathy.

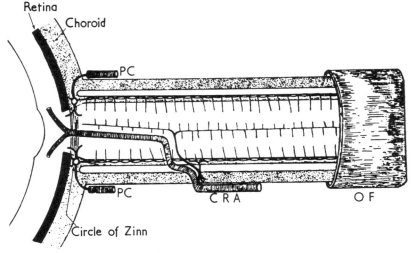

Fig. 13.1. Vascular supply of the optic nerve.

PC: posterior ciliary artery
CRA: central retinal artery
OF: Optic foramen.
(After *Wolff—Anatomy of the Eye and Orbit.* London, H. K. Lewis).

Ischaemic Papillopathy (Ischaemic optic neuropathy)

Occlusion of the arteries supplying the anterior portion of the optic nerve and the optic disc produces a clinical picture different from central retinal occlusion, though blindness of abrupt onset is common to both. The condition is referred to as 'ischaemic papillopathy'. This is commonly due to giant-cell or temporal arteritis, and occasionally to arteriosclerosis, and affects elderly patients in particular. Abrupt loss of vision over a period of a few hours or less is the presenting symptom, and total loss of vision in one or both eyes usual. Recovery of vision is rare. The visual loss is often bilateral in giant-cell arteritis, but it may be unilateral in arteriosclerosis.

Ophthalmic examination reveals a pale and moderately swollen disc, sometimes accompanied by a few small linear haemorrhages and cottonwool patches near the disc (*Fig.* 13.2). The pallor of the optic disc is the striking feature, and is due to ischaemia, in marked contrast to the pink or red swelling of the papilloedema caused by raised intracranial pressure, except when the latter is subsiding into consecutive optic atrophy. The retinal vessels may appear relatively normal, especially in giant-cell arteritis, though some arterial narrowing and irregularity of lumen may be seen if the papillopathy is arteriosclerotic in origin. The appearance is quite unlike that of central retinal artery occlusion, with its

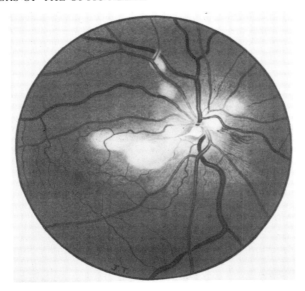

Fig. 13.2. Optic fundus of ischaemic papillopathy in giant-cell arteritis (an unusually florid example).

general retinal pallor, narrowed arteries and 'cherry red spot' at the macular (*see Fig.* 11.2). The ischaemic swelling of the optic nerve gradually subsides to be replaced by optic atrophy which is permanent. Although blindness is often total in one or both eyes, a small portion of the peripheral field may be retained. In some instances central vision may remain relatively intact if the macula receives an alternative retinal blood supply.

Giant-cell (temporal) arteritis is the commonest cause of ischaemic papillopathy and occurs almost exclusively in the elderly. The clinical manifestations are largely caused by gradual arterial occlusion and include sudden blindness and less commonly cerebral or cardiac infarction, and such widespread symptoms as general weakness, polymyalgia and loss of weight. The larger and medium sized arteries are primarily affected in an irregular and patchy fashion, though the renal arteries appear to be rarely involved, which is probably a factor in the usually favourable outcome of the disorder, except for blindness. The histological features are chiefly in the media, with disintegration of the internal elastic lamina, and cellular infiltration with mono-nuclear and plasma cells, and occasional polymorphs and eosinophils, but the striking feature is the presence of multinucleated giant cells. The intima shows diffuse thickening and the lumen may be reduced to a slit (*Fig.* 13.3).

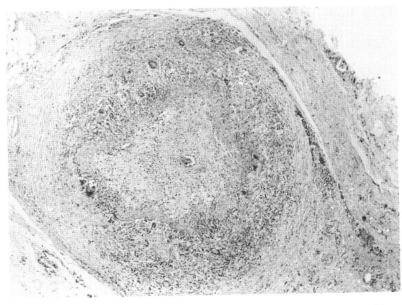

Fig. 13.3. Section of temporal artery in giant-cell arteritis (granulomatous arteritis with giant cells).

From the clinical aspect involvement of the temporal and occipital arteries of the scalp, and of the ophthalmic branch of the internal carotid artery reign supreme. There is usually an initial period of severe headache, or pain in the temporal region of the scalp, which may last some days or even weeks. The pain may spread widely to the occipital region, face, jaws and tongue. The superficial temporal arteries are often swollen, nodular and tender, and pulsation may be diminished or absent (*Fig.* 13.4). Loss of vision of abrupt onset, or occasionally more gradual over a period of a few hours, is the striking feature. In a minority of cases, premonitory visual symptoms, such as temporary obscuration of vision or visual hallucinations (coloured lights or even more organized patterns) may precede total visual loss. One or both eyes may be affected, the second eye often becoming involved within a few days. The severe headache may subside soon after the onset of blindness.

Diplopia due to a 6th or partial 3rd nerve palsy occurs in a small proportion of cases of giant-cell arteritis, and may mimic the clinical features of subarachnoid haemorrhage due to an intracranial aneurysm. This diplopia may precede the onset of blindness and hence is an added indication for urgent steroid therapy. The ocular palsies have a better prognosis than loss of vision, and often recover within a few months.

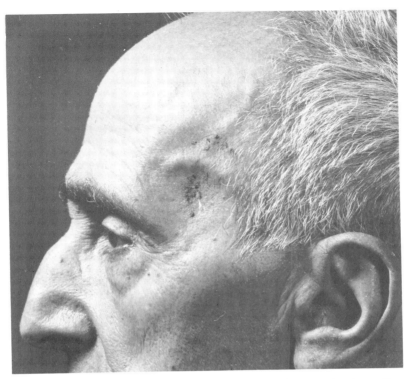

Fig. 13.4. Swollen and nodular superficial temporal artery in giant-cell arteritis.

The visual loss is usually total in one or both eyes, but vision is occasionally retained in a small portion of the field, usually peripheral. In rare instances central vision remains relatively intact, causing a 'tubular' visual field, due to the presence of an alternative blood supply to the macula via a cilioretinal artery.

Although the visual loss is ischaemic in origin the classic appearance of central retinal arterial occlusion is very uncommon. The ophthalmoscopic features are usually those of ischaemic papillopathy as described previously. The severity of the visual loss is often much greater than the visible changes in the optic fundus.

Post-mortem examination in one personal case showed severe arteritis involving the ophthalmic, ciliary and central retinal arteries outside the globe, with no evidence of involvement of the arteries in the eye itself. Location of the ischaemic damage to the papilla and anterior portion of the optic nerve appears to be the main cause of the visual loss, with consequent ischaemic papillopathy.

The erythrocyte sedimentation rate (ESR) is almost always raised, and is a simple and rapid test affording confirmatory evidence of the disorder. Biopsy of the tortuous and tender superficial temporal artery should also be undertaken, as it usually affords undisputable evidence of the diagnosis.

Urgent treatment, even before biopsy, with high dose steroids (prednisolone 60 mg daily) is indicated, and there seems little doubt that this can prevent the onset of blindness, if administered early enough; once vision is lost recovery on steroid therapy does not occur. If the sight of one eye has already been lost, immediate steroid therapy (even intravenously) may prevent involvement of the second eye. Early diagnosis before the onset of blindness is thus imperative.

Visual failure may occur when the patient is on steroid therapy, usually within 10 days of the start of treatment, and it seems likely that the arterial supply of the optic nerve and retina is at that time at a critical level, and that therapy was instituted too late to prevent blindness, a case of *post hoc* rather than *propter hoc*. In one patient of the present writer, a man of 74 years, prednisolone therapy was instituted 2 weeks after the onset of unilateral blindness. Seven days later vision began to deteriorate in the remaining eye, but loss of vision was limited to the inferior portion of the visual field, without involvement of central vision, so that the patient was left with useful vision in one eye (*Fig.* 13.5). Such arrest does not occur during the natural course of the disorder, and must be attributed to steroid therapy.

Giant-cell arteritis appears to be a self-limiting disorder, with a tendency to burn itself out over a period of many months. It is not commonly fatal, but often leaves blindness in its trail.

Occlusion of the central retinal artery and central retinal veins is discussed elsewhere (Chapter 11).

OPTIC NEURITIS (RETROBULBAR NEURITIS)

Unilateral optic or retrobulbar neuritis is one of the cardinal features of disseminated (multiple) sclerosis, and due to demyelination of the optic nerve. This is very rare in the elderly, being most common under the age of 45 years. Loss of vision of gradual onset occurs over a period of a few hours or days, and a central scotoma with full peripheral field is usual. The optic fundus may be entirely normal or the optic disc slightly or moderately swollen (papillitis). Recovery of vision is usual over the succeeding few weeks, but pallor of the disc (optic atrophy) is a common sequel.

Bilateral retrobulbar neuritis is much less common in disseminated sclerosis, either two separate episodes, or rarely the simultaneous affection of both eyes. Leber's hereditary optic atrophy is bilateral, but is rarely encountered after the age of 30 years. Bilateral retrobulbar neuritis may also be of toxic origin, and even occur in the elderly, but is uncommon. Methyl alcohol, ethyl alcohol, tobacco and chloroquine can cause bilateral visual failure.

Methyl alcohol is a vicious retinal and optic nerve poison. Ingestion may be followed by vomiting, prostration and coma, sometimes accompanied by convulsions, and soon followed by bilateral blindness. The latter may be total or consist of bilateral central scotomatous defects, and there is rarely any significant recovery of vision. One personal case followed ingestion of methyl alcohol by a pharmacist in mistake for ethyl alcohol as an aperitif, and a second case followed ingestion of after-shave lotion by an alcoholic patient.

There seems little doubt that on occasion excessive alcoholic intake, especially of spirits, and often associated with excessive tobacco smoking, may cause bilateral retrobulbar neuritis, perhaps more likely in a confirmed alcoholic patient. The visual defects, though central scotomatous in type, are not typical of tobacco amblyopia per se. Vision may recover almost completely following abstension from alcohol.

Tobacco amblyopia is relatively uncommon, and tends to occur in middle-aged or elderly pipe smokers. It is rare in cigarette smokers and in women. Excessive alcoholic consumption seems to increase the incidence and severity of the visual loss. The hallmark of tobacco amblyopia is the visual field defect (Fig. 13.6): bilateral centro-caecal scotomas, horizontally oval with sloping edges, and small dense nuclei inside the scotoma. The earliest defect is a small scotoma to the temporal side of fixation, which gradually spreads laterally to involve fixation. The optic discs are normal, at least in the early stages, and severe optic atrophy does not appear. Tobacco amblyopia is more likely to appear if there is a deficiency of vitamin B_{12}, as in Addisonian (pernicious) anaemia, and the visual defect may clear fairly rapidly on vitamin B_{12} therapy with cobalamin, even if the patient continues smoking. It may be that the small amount of cyanide in tobacco smoke is a factor. Vitamin B_{12} avidly takes up and detoxicates cyanide and a deficiency of vitamin B_{12} may leave free cyanide. Massive B_{12} therapy by intramuscular injection is indicated (cobalamin (Neocytamen) 100 μg weekly).

Bilateral retrobulbar neuritis is a rare, but well documented, manifestation of Addisonian (pernicious) anaemia, and of its associated subacute combined degeneration of the cord, where there is a deficiency of vitamin B_{12}. The early institution of treatment by B_{12} therapy can abolish the symptoms of both disorders.

Optic atrophy is a rare complication of diabetes mellitus, usually in elderly patients with long-standing diabetes. Little is known about its causation, whether nutritional or ischaemic, but it is quite separate from diabetic retinopathy. In young diabetics the condition may be hereditary and allied to Leber's disease.

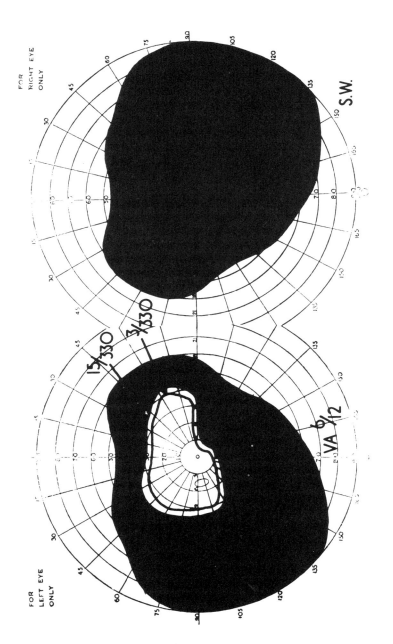

Fig. 13.5. Visual fields of case of giant-cell arteritis, with arrest of loss of vision in second eye on steroid therapy.

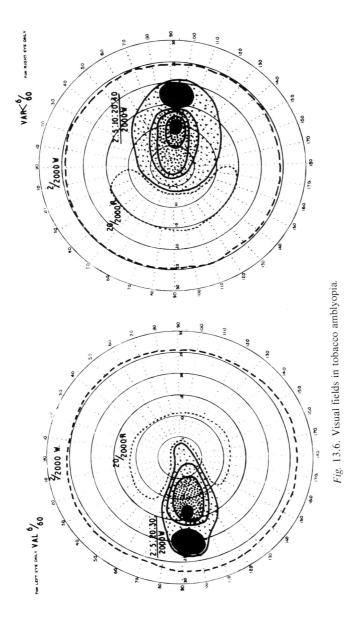

Fig. 13.6. Visual fields in tobacco amblyopia.

Bilateral retrobulbar neuritis has also been recorded in carcinomatosis, without direct involvement of the optic nerve by metastatic tumour cells, and possibly due to secondary malnutrition or vitamin deficiency.

OPTIC NERVE COMPRESSION

Compression of the optic nerve occurs at all ages, including the elderly, and is considered here as a clinical entity, though there are individual differences in clinical expression between the various compressing agents. Although compression may occur with the orbit, by tumours or granulomas and usually accompanied by exophthalmos, the vast majority of cases are due to intracranial involvement of the nerve, chiefly by meningiomas or aneurysms. Such compression may continue for months, and even years, with little in evidence except progressive unilateral, and later bilateral, visual failure and increasing pallor of the optic disc. Headache and other symptoms may be absent in the early stages, so that the diagnosis may not be made until the condition is well advanced, and even inoperable. Successful treatment depends above all on early diagnosis, which in turn depends on a detailed and diligent clinical history and examination. The subject therefore needs careful scrutiny, including the history of visual failure, examination of the visual fields, acuity and optic fundi, as well as a complete general medical and neurological examination. Most important of all is the necessity to bear in mind the possibility of optic nerve compression in cases of progressive unilateral visual failure with little ophthalmoscopic abnormality apart from increasing optic disc pallor.

Meningiomas are probably the commonest cause of unilateral optic nerve compression. Those arising intracranially from the anterior clinoid or medial portion of the sphenoidal ridge, tuberculum sellae and olfactory groove are particularly situated to compress the optic nerve, unilaterally in the early stages (*Figs.* 13.7 *and* 13.8). Tumours of the optic nerve itself are much less common, and include meningiomas of the optic nerve sheath, and gliomas of the nerve itself. The latter usually present in childhood, but meningiomas of the nerve occur at a later age, and even in the elderly. These meningiomas may arise from the arachnoid surrounding the optic nerve in the orbit, and spread posteriorly through the optic foramen, or from a sphenoidal ridge (medial third) meningioma extending forward to the orbit, in each case forming a dumb-bell tumour, partly intracranial and partly intra-orbital, and enlarging the optic foramen; this is visible by radiography. These meningiomas are often encapsulated and excisable, but occasionally spread widely as a meningioma *en plaque,* in which case exophthalmos and ocular palsy are to be expected in addition to loss of vision caused by compression of the optic nerve.

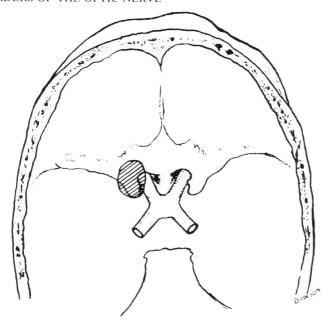

Fig. 13.7. Diagram of small meningioma arising from anterior clinoid process and compressing optic nerve.

An *intracranial aneurysm* suitably placed may gradually expand and compress one optic nerve (*Fig.* 13.9), often without any history of subarachnoid haemorrhage, and sometimes even without pain or headache. The aneurysmal nature of the compression may therefore be entirely unsuspected on clinical grounds, and only be demonstrated on arteriography or CT scan. Aneurysms arising from the anterior cerebral and anterior communicating arteries, or from the terminal portion of the internal carotid artery as it passes upwards lateral to the optic chiasm, are particularly sited to cause optic nerve compression.

A pituitary adenoma, commonly chromophobe, may first cause symptoms in the elderly. Compression of the optic chiasm is the usual method of presentation, with consequent bitemporal hemianopic defects, but occasionally lateral expansion compresses one optic nerve in the initial stages. There may be clinical signs of hypopituitarism. Other less common causes of optic nerve compression include metastasis from a distant carcinoma (breast, lung or gastrointestinal) and a tortuous arteriosclerotic internal carotid artery.

The clinical features of optic nerve compression may be so undramatic, with unilateral visual loss as the sole symptom, and little or

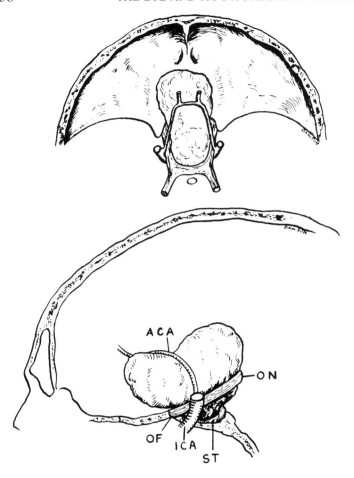

Fig. 13.8. Diagram of large meningioma lying between optic nerves and displacing optic chiasm backwards (10 years after onset of unilateral visual failure).

ACA: anterior cerebral artery
ON: optic nerve
OF: optic foramen
ICA: internal carotid artery
ST: sella turcica.

no pain or headache, that the examiner may be lulled into inactivity, which can be fatal to the patient. Progressive unilateral visual failure is the essential clinical feature. It may be so unobtrusive that it is not noticed by the patient until he accidentally closes his good eye, to find

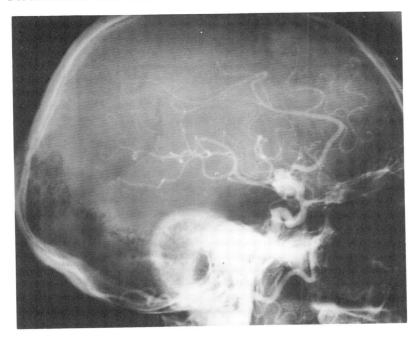

Fig. 13.9. Arteriogram showing aneurysm of terminal portion of internal carotid artery, compressing optic nerve and optic chiasm.

that the other eye is virtually blind, in which case the loss of vision may be regarded as of sudden onset, and vascular or demyelinating disorders considered likely. In fact such a history suggests a previously unnoticed visual loss of gradual onset.

Visual failure may be of several months' or even years' duration (except in metastatic involvement) before the patient presents himself. Headache is not a prominent feature in the early stages, except in some cases of intracranial aneurysm, but even aneurysmal compression may be entirely painless.

The visual field defect is of paramount importance. A central scotoma may be a feature in the early stages, thus mimicking retrobulbar neuritis, but the defect soon spreads to the periphery in one or other segment of the field, leaving a peripheral rim of intact vision, which is eventually lost, leaving total unilateral blindness (*Fig.* 13.10). In some cases the visual loss starts in the periphery and gradually spreads across the field like a curtain. The importance of gradual and progressive extension of the field loss cannot be overstressed.

A defect in the upper temporal field of the opposite eye may appear

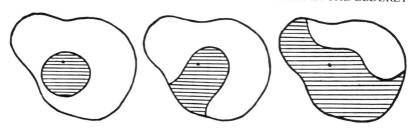

Fig. 13.10. Diagram of progressive field loss in compression of right optic nerve by meningioma (over a period of several months).

later, due to involvement of the crossed nasal fibres from the contralateral optic nerve. The lower nasal fibres, representing the contralateral upper visual field, pass slightly forwards, before joining the optic tract (*Fig.* 13.11). Unilateral blindness in association with an upper temporal field defect in the contralateral eye is almost diagnostic of a compressive lesion.

The optic fundus may be entirely normal in the early stages of the optic nerve compression, even up to a year or more after the onset of symptoms, which may encourage a fatal 'wait-and-see' attitude. Eventually pallor of the optic disc gradually supervenes, terminating in optic atrophy. The blood vessels of the optic nerve are involved in the compressive process, and ischaemia of the optic nerve is a potential factor in neural damage. Retrograde demyelination between the point of compression in the optic nerve and the retina is also a factor in the production of optic atrophy.

In the early stages of compression there is no evidence of increased intracranial pressure, but this may supervene later, with the appearance of papilloedema in the contralateral eye (Foster–Kennedy syndrome). This occurs with tumours rather than aneurysms, and is indicative of a more serious prognosis.

Additional clinical features may include anosmia, from a meningioma of the olfactory groove, and ipsilateral exophthalmos from spread of a meningioma into the orbit, often along the optic nerve sheath. A bruit audible over the eye is extremely rare, even in cases of aneurysm. Clinical signs of hypopituitarism, such as smooth skin, facial pallor, loss of hair over the face, axillae and pubes, and amenorrhoea or impotence are suggestive of a chromophobe adenoma of the pituitary. Craniopharyngiomas rarely present in the elderly.

A meningioma, the commonest cause of optic nerve compression, can often be completely excised neurosurgically in the early stages, but later expansion may involve the anterior cerebral and internal carotid arteries, making complete neurosurgical removal wellnigh impossible.

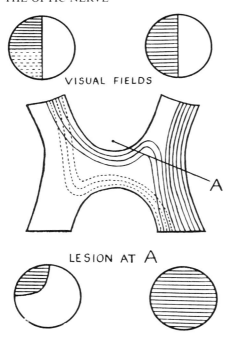

VISUAL FIELDS

LESION AT A

Fig. 13.11. Probable course of crossed nasal fibres of optic nerve in optic chiasm, and field defect due to compression at A (posterior extremity of optic nerve). continuous line represents lower nasal fibres, and interrupted line represents upper nasal fibres.

An anterior communicating aneurysm may be clipped, or even excised in some cases.

Traumatic optic atrophy occurs in a small proportion of closed head injuries, and due to indirect injury to the optic nerve, is usually unilateral and often unaccompanied by fracture of the skull or optic foramen. The skull impact is usually supra-orbital in site and severe in degree. Loss of vision of one eye is noticed on recovery from consciousness, and optic atrophy gradually supervenes during the succeeding few weeks. Complete unilateral blindness is usual and permanent, but traumatic damage to the optic nerve is sometimes partial, with loss of part of the visual field, in which case some recovery of vision is possible within the next few weeks.

SUMMARY

This chapter is primarily concerned with the clinical aspects of lesions of the optic nerve, so that investigations have not been discussed in detail.

Straight X-rays of the skull, sella and optic foramina are carried out in appropriate cases, but the role of air pictures and arteriography has receded in the case of space-occupying lesions, to be replaced by computerized tomography, because of its safety and the information it conveys. Special cuts in the plane of the optic nerve are required, and in many cases this virtually establishes the definitive diagnosis. Angiography is still performed if there is reason to suspect an aneurysm or other vascular pathology, or where the neurosurgeon needs to know the precise course of vessels to avoid damage in certain operations.

ACKNOWLEDGEMENTS

I am grateful to Dr John Meadows for constructive criticism, and also to Mr A. H. Prentice of the Photography Department of the National Hospital, Queen Square, London, for the drawing of *Figure* 13.1 and for processing the illustrations.

FURTHER READING

Meadows S. P. (1949) *Proc. R. Soc. Med.* **42**, 1017.
Meadows S. P. (1966) *Proc. R. Soc. Med.* **59**, 329.
Parsons-Smith B. G. (1952) *Br. J. Ophthalmol.* **36**, 615.
Parsons-Smith B. G. (1959) *Br. J. Ophthalmol.* **43**, 204.
Russell R. W. R. (1959) *Q. J. Med.* **28**, 471.

14. NEURO-OPHTHALMOLOGY
Bryan Ashworth

This chapter reviews the diagnostic significance of the pupil, the management of ocular myasthenia, and some cortical disorders of vision.

THE PUPIL

The pupils tend to diminish in size as age advances. Careful observation of normal people reveals differences in diameter of up to 1 mm (Meyer, 1947).

Oval pupils may be attributable to cerebral vascular disease and are sometimes seen as a transient feature during recovery from brainstem lesions (Fisher, 1980). The shape is presumably due to interruption of motor innervation to segments of the iris. The same explanation may apply to the ectopic pupils described by Kinnier Wilson in brainstem disease (Wilson, 1906). Oval pupils in cerebral vascular disease indicate a poor prognosis.

When the pupil is smaller on one side and the palpebral fissure on that side is narrower a lesion of the sympathetic innervation will be suspected. Horner's syndrome due to disease of the central nervous system is likely to be associated with vertigo, sensory deficit, and other signs localizing to the brainstem or upper spinal cord. The sympathetic pathway may also be interrupted in its peripheral course by tumour, thoracotomy, and injuries to the neck or brachial plexus.

In the elderly patient Horner's syndrome may be associated with fibrotic changes around the common carotid artery (Goldhammer, 1982). Alternating Horner's syndrome is sometimes seen with lesions of the cervical cord. Usually the disorder is central but it has been attributed to dural adhesions after injury (Ottomo and Heimburger, 1980). Reversed Horner's syndrome due to sympathetic irritation is shown as a dilated pupil associated with excessive unilateral sweating and lid retraction. It is met with in patients with tumours in the neck, apical tuberculosis, or after surgical operations on the neck.

The Argyll–Robertson pupil is now seen infrequently but most often in the elderly when it is the consequence of past syphilitic infection. It may

143

be mimicked by diabetes mellitus (Smith et al., 1978) and by lesions in the pineal region—usually tumours which are often associated with paresis of vertical gaze (Seybold et al., 1971). The normal range of upward gaze diminishes as age advances (Chamberlain, 1971).

The Holmes—Adie syndrome is unlikely to develop in old age but may lead to difficulty in diagnosis. In a typical patient one pupil is larger than the other, unreactive to light, and slow to respond in convergence. Some or all of the tendon jerks are absent. It has been shown that there is destruction of the ciliary ganglion (Rüttner, 1947; Harriman and Garland, 1968), as was predicted from the constriction produced by local mecholyl (Scheie, 1940). The clinical features at various stages cannot all be explained by loss of the ciliary ganglion. Isolated segments of the iris may lose their nerve supply; this would explain the irregularity of the pupil. Sprouting of nerves may lead to imperfect re-innervation and be combined with cholinergic hypersensitivity (Thompson, 1977; Bell and Thompson, 1978; Bourgon et al., 1978; Thompson, 1978; Wirtschafter et al., 1978; Loewenfeld and Thompson, 1981).

OCULAR MYASTHENIA

Double vision and ptosis are common presenting symptoms in myasthenia but the peculiar vulnerability of the external ocular muscles has not been explained. More than half of a group of these patients go on to develop generalized myasthenia, the majority within two years (Bever et al., 1981). In a significant proportion variously estimated at 20–40 per cent, the clinical features remain confined to the ocular muscles and the orbicularis oculi. Ocular myasthenia has a good prognosis but is often difficult to treat.

Myasthenia may begin in old age, and I have seen it develop in a man of 92. It is a rare disease affecting about 1 in 50000 of the population. The aetiology is uncertain, although evidence of autoimmune disorder is accumulating. It is sometimes associated with pernicious anaemia, systemic lupus, or thyroid disease (Simpson, 1960).

At the myoneural junction acetylcholine allows the nerve impulse to pass to the muscle receptor. It has been known for many years that neostigmine and pyridostigmine are anti-cholinesterase drugs and therefore promote the action of acetylcholine. It remained uncertain whether the disturbance in myasthenia is pre- or post-synaptic. New light has been shed on this by the demonstration that patients with generalized myasthenia have a high titre of acetylcholine-receptor-antibody in their serum (Ito et al., 1978). This provided further support for the autoimmune hypothesis and led the way to a diagnostic test for the disease. Acetylcholine-receptor-antibody shows a high specificity for myasthenia. The titre has been found to be increased in most patients with the generalized type of myasthenia but less frequently in ocular myasthenia (Vincent and Newsom-Davis, 1980).

Suspicion of myasthenia will be aroused when there is a painless ptosis or limitation of eye movement with diplopia; it is common to find weakness of the orbicularis oculi muscles as well. The features are often asymmetrical, sometimes unilateral, and characteristically fluctuate from minute to minute.

Confirmation of the diagnosis may be obtained by the response to intravenous edrophonium chloride (Tensilon). Subjective improvement is of no value, but resolution of the signs may be striking and often cannot be maintained subsequently with drugs such as pyridostigmine.

Special caution is needed in those with unstable cardiac arrhythmias or heart failure; it is wise to have the patient lying on a couch. The response is seen in about a minute and fades in a few minutes (*Fig.* 14.1). This test is positive in most cases of myasthenia but if negative is worth repeating. A negative test may suggest ocular myopathy (Osserman and Genkins, 1966).

If the diagnosis of myasthenia is confirmed it is helpful to obtain a chest radiograph, erythrocyte sedimentation rate (ESR), serum antinuclear factor estimation, and thyroid function tests. Collagen diseases and thyroid disorders are commoner with patients with myasthenia than in the general population. Special chest radiography such as tomography is usually unhelpful unless plain radiographs show enlargement of the thymus.

Thymectomy has been carried out for many years; the gland is often enlarged in generalized myasthenia. In most cases there is hyperplasia; a small proportion show malignant change. The identification of acetyl-choline-receptor antibody has provided a rationale for thymectomy, and removal of the gland is now usually advised in patients with generalized disease at an early stage.

Treatment is difficult, and the patient with ocular myasthenia may be better without it. Diplopia can be relieved by the occlusion of one eye. It is worth a trial of pyridostigmine 60 mg given twice daily and increased to 3 or 4 tablets daily. Abdominal colic can be relieved with propantheline 15 mg, which is usually needed if the dose of pyri-dostigmine is greater than 180 mg daily. A few patients obtain complete relief with this regime, and they should continue with it, but in most there is little improvement. Sometimes the condition is made worse—for example, if ptosis is relieved and diplopia unmasked. A higher dose of pyridostigmine often fails to give control; it may be better to abandon the drugs when large doses are needed or unwanted effects produced.

The use of mechanical devices such as ptosis props to support the eyelid in patients with ptosis is not usually satisfactory. Surgical operations on the lids should be avoided in these patients.

Corticosteroid therapy may induce a remission in myasthenia, but

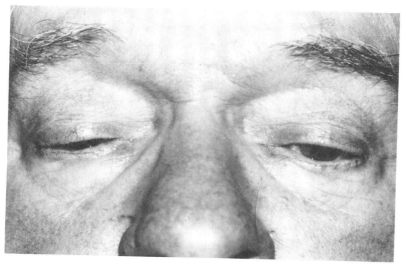

a

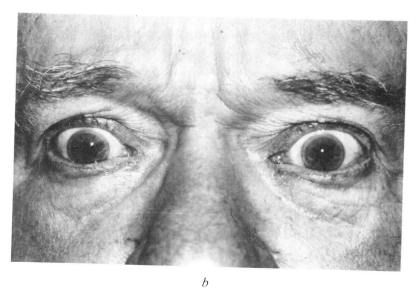

b

Fig. 14.1. Ocular Myasthenia:
a. Bilateral and asymmetrical ptosis
b. Response to intravenous Tensilon.

difficulties arise because high dosage is needed and withdrawal leads to relapse. The patient illustrated in *Fig.* 14.1 did not respond to a course of prednisolone 100 mg on alternate days. He was then given methyl-prednisolone 1 g daily intravenously; this produced complete remission, but within a week of stopping the therapy he had relapsed. There is a risk of temporary worsening of the myasthenia when large doses of corticosteroid are given, and this should only be done in hospital. Out-patient treatment begins with much smaller doses such as prednisolone 10 mg daily. The results are variable and the unwanted effects troublesome. In general, it seems better to avoid corticosteroids in ocular myasthenia.

Immunosuppression, plasmapheresis, and thymectomy, which are used in generalized myasthenia, are not recommended in the ocular type. This is because all these measures carry risks which are not generally considered justified in a benign disorder.

It has been pointed out that it is impossible to predict at an early stage the course of myasthenia. Confirmation that it remains confined to the ocular muscles is only possible after observation over several years. Patients with ocular myasthenia have a normal life span. Remission may occur spontaneously, but this is unusual in the elderly.

THE CHIASMA AND POSTERIOR VISUAL PATHWAY

Diagnosis in this area has been improved by new techniques in radiology and particularly by computerized tomography (CT). Chiasmal lesions lead to impaired acuity and a field defect, classically a bitemporal hemianopia, but often asymmetrical or atypical in the early stages. Pituitary tumours which give rise to this are large, often of the chromophobe type, and have usually caused erosion of the sella on a plain radiograph. Similar visual effects may be due to suprasellar meningioma, craniopharyngioma (Russell and Pennybacker, 1961), or aneurysm (Raymond and Tew, 1978); any of these may present in old age. Advances in surgery and the use of the operating microscope have improved results. There is a trend towards removal of pituitary tumours by the trans-sphenoidal route.

Visual Disturbance in Post-Chiasmal Lesions

It is characteristic of post-chiasmal disorders that the patient is unaware of the visual deficit and finds out about it by colliding with an object in the blind field rather than by sensing it. A distinction may be made between lesions of the primary visual pathway from chiasma to occipital cortex associated with a field defect, and disorders of the visual association areas or corpus callosum which disturb higher cortical visual function. Often the same pathological process will involve both areas. With unilateral lesions behind the lateral geniculate body, the pupillary reactions, visual acuity and optic fundi are normal. It is important to realize that objective signs are often lacking; this should not lead to the assumption that the condition is psychological.

An estimate of the neuronal loss from the visual cortex with age based on 24 subjects aged 20–80 years showed that at 80 years the loss was almost half (Devaney and Johnson, 1980). Some progress in the understanding of cortical defects of vision has come from case reports of individual patients with demonstration of the lesion by CT scan, study of groups of patients with similar lesions, psychometric observations, and animal experiments. The CT scan depends on tissue density and is helpful both in location of the lesion and in giving some indication of the probable pathology.

Lesions of the Posterior Visual Pathway

Three case summaries will illustrate the correlation of clinical and radiological features.

Case 1: A woman of 53 years reported a sensation of flashing lights on the left side. The next day she had difficulty in reading and found that she was missing out words or letters. She tended to bump into things on the left and was lethargic.

Examination showed a complete left homonymous hemianopia, with BP 230/110, and no other signs. The haemoglobin was 10·8 g per cent and the red cells normochromic and normocytic, with the ESR 65 mm/h. Clinical examination did not reveal any evidence of tumour. The CT scan (*Fig.* 14.2a) showed a mass in the right occipital area which enhanced with contrast. Intravenous pyelography indicated a left renal tumour and the abdominal CT scan showed that this had extended outside the renal capsule (*Fig.* 14.2b). The diagnosis was hypernephroma with cerebral metastasis.

Case 2: A woman of 64 was admitted with a history of persistent and generalized headache for a week. Examination showed a complete left homonymous hemianopia. The unenhanced CT scan demonstrated areas of high density in the right occipital lobe indicative of haemorrhage (*Fig.* 14.3). The headache settled, and the haematoma subsided spontaneously, but the field defect remained. The diagnosis was hypertension complicated by cerebral haemorrhage.

Case 3: A man of 57 years reported a visual sensation like sparks on the right side, associated with tingling in the right arm and leg and numbness of the right side of the face. Examination showed an upper quadrant homonymous hemianopia to the right, right hemianalgesia, and increased tendon jerks on the right. Both plantar responses were extensor. BP 140/90. The CT scan showed a focal low density area in the left paramedian occipital zone corresponding with the occipital cortex. It did not enhance with contrast (*Fig.* 14.4). A diagnosis of partial infarction of the left occipital lobe was made. The field loss remained unchanged, but the other symptoms cleared.

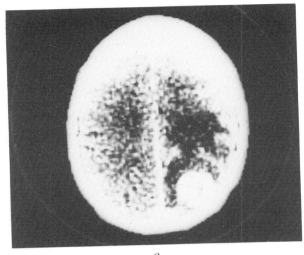

a

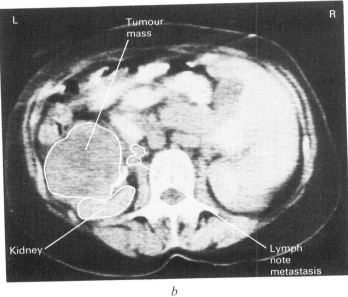

b

Fig. 14.2.
a. CT scan with enhancement showing dense lesion in right occipito-parietal area
and altered density of surrounding tissues attributed to oedema.
b. CT scan of abdomen showing large left kidney with tumour mass outside the
capsule.

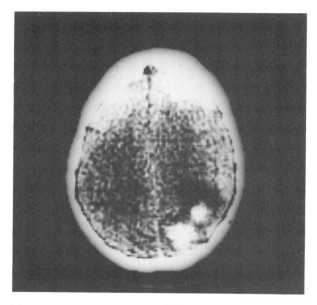

Fig. 14.3. Intracerebral haemorrhage: CT scan without enhancement showing irregular areas of high density in right occipital lobe with surrounding oedema.

VISUAL PERCEPTION

The importance of the left cerebral hemisphere in relation to speech has been appreciated for many years. Visuo-spatial information is processed mainly in the right hemisphere. Localization of the lesion which has caused a disorder of visual perception is of importance in clinical diagnosis, but may also contribute to understanding of the inter-relationship of speech, writing, and visual function.

Disorders of Visual Perception

There is an inability to interpret what is seen and integrate it with past experience. This may be part of a generalized cerebral disorder accompanied by dementia; then no useful analysis is possible. The rare examples of isolated defects can be studied and several syndromes defined.

Visual object agnosia is an inability to recognize an object by visual channels, although it is seen, and may be identified by touch. The disturbance is usually part of a diffuse cerebral disorder and is often accompanied by dysphasia and mental confusion. It cannot be attributed to localized lesions (Critchley, 1964).

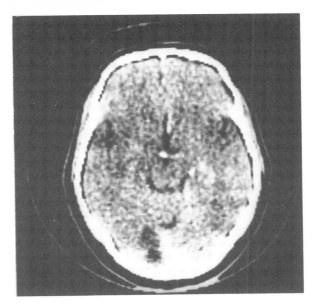

Fig. 14.4. Cerebral infarction: Enhanced scan showing paramedian area of reduced density. Left occipital lobe.

Prosopagnosia or inability to recognize faces that were previously familiar is homonymous hemianopia.

Case 4: A man of 67 had been treated for systemic hypertension but therapy was allowed to lapse. A few weeks before he was seen a sudden episode occurred and was followed by difficulty in reading and writing. Things were seen more clearly on the right side. He was unable to recognize his wife or his friends from their appearance and had similar difficulty in identifying people seen on television. Examination showed an alert man with normal speech and BP 240/120. Confrontation tests revealed an inferior quadrantic left homonymous hemianopia. The corrected visual acuity and the optic discs were normal. The neurological examination was otherwise negative. The CT scan showed evidence of bilateral cerebral atrophy which was marked in the area of the occipital lobes (*Fig.* 14.5). Recent occipital lobe infarction on a basis of basilar artery ischaemia seemed likely. His condition has remained unchanged over the past three years.

In these cases the patient may not be able to recognize himself seen in a mirror. Matching of photographs may be possible. Cases of prosopagnosia which have come to autopsy have all shown bilateral occipital lobe disease but the right occipito-temporal area is particularly

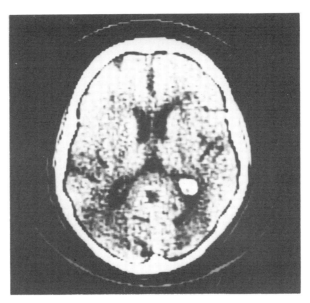

Fig. 14.5. Prosopagnosia. Cerebral infarction: CT scan showing slight ventricular dilatation and subcortical areas of reduced density of both occipital lobes.

important, and it has been claimed that a single lesion here may cause the defect (Pevzner et al., 1962; Meadows, 1974a; Whiteley and Warrington, 1977; Damasio et al., 1982; Malone et al., 1982).

Simultanagnosia: The patient who looks at a picture, recognizes the detail but fails to appreciate the meaning as a whole or is slow to do so. Words are only understood by spelling out the individual letters. The disorder is most often associated with a lesion of the inferior part of the left occipital lobe (Kinsbourne and Warrington, 1963).

Achromatopsia: Inability to interpret colours is sometimes found in patients with prosopagnosia and may be unilateral. It has been reported with lesions of the right occipital lobe and within that lobe relates particularly to the antero-inferior part (Meadows, 1974b; Albert et al., 1975; Green and Lessell, 1977; Brazis et al., 1981).

Visual neglect: A patient with intact field of vision may neglect objects on one side. This has usually been attributed to a parietal lobe lesion. Neglect of things to the left side is much commoner than to the right. While it is not disputed that the right parietal lobe may be affected in such cases evidence accumulates that lesions in other parts of the brain may give rise to unilateral neglect.

Visual neglect may be demonstrated by the behaviour of the patient, the failure to recognize simultaneous movements of fingers on opposite sides while each is detected singly, by asking him to draw simple objects or patterns and to bisect a line drawn on a piece of paper (when the division will be unequal).

Neglect may be due to defective arousal, attention, or action. Experimentally in the monkey it can be shown that hemispatial neglect may be produced by lesions in the opposite frontal lobe, thalamus, or mesencephalic reticular formation. In some instances there is no lesion of sensory pathways and the disorder is classified as motor neglect (Heilman and Valenstein, 1979).

In human subjects profound contralateral neglect may be associated with haemorrhage in the right thalamus. This may be due to interruption of fibres passing from the reticular formation to the parietal lobe (Watson and Heilman, 1979). Haemorrhage in the left thalamus causes dysphasia but neglect may also be demonstrated to the right side (Alexander and LoVerme, 1980).

Acquired dyslexia: Difficulty in reading due to acquired disease may be associated with dysphasia, dysgraphia, and right homonymous hemianopia which point to a lesion of the left hemisphere. Particular interest attaches to the rather unusual finding of dyslexia without agraphia. Sometimes this arises without a field defect.

Case 5: A man of 60 was seen because of difficulty in reading. There was a history of episodes of mental confusion and then a major myocardial infarction with disorder of cardiac rhythm which was controlled with a pacemaker. On the following day he could not read and had some difficulty in finding words. He was able to write but could not read what he had written in normal script. Examination later showed a persistent right homonymous hemianopia with dyslexia, normal speech and no other disability. He said that he recognized colours but not their associations. For example, he no longer regarded red as a sign of danger.

The CT scan showed a low density lesion in the left parieto-occipital area which did not enhance (*Fig.* 14.6). It was attributed to infarction during a phase of low cerebral perfusion provoked by cardiovascular collapse.

The condition of alexia without agraphia is usually due to a lesion of the left angular gyrus or its connections as was demonstrated in this patient. It may be due to trauma, vascular disease or tumour. It can be classified as a disconnection syndrome when the lesion is subcortical and interrupts fibres in the visual association area or corpus callosum (Geschwind, 1965; Greenblatt, 1973; L'Hermitte and Beauvois, 1973; Cohen et al., 1976; Skipkin et al., 1981).

CONCLUSION AND SUMMARY

Lesions of the primary visual pathway may be recognized from the nature of the field defect. The CT scan is helpful in localizing the lesion

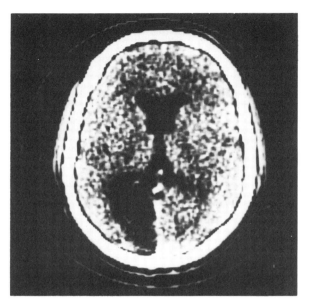

Fig. 14.6: Alexia without dysgraphia. Cerebral infarction: CT scan showing moderate dilatation of cerebral ventricles with extensive area of reduced density in left occipito-parietal area.

and may also give an indication of the pathology. Disorders of visual perception are not always associated with a field defect. Visual agnosia cannot be attributed to a localized cerebral lesion. Prosopagnosia is usually due to bilateral occipital lobe disease and the right occipito-temporal area is particularly important. Simultanagnosia relates to the inferior part of the left occipital lobe. Visual neglect is not always due to a lesion of the parietal lobe. Acquired dyslexia without agraphia is usually due to a lesion of the left angular gyrus or its connections.

ACKNOWLEDGEMENTS

I wish to thank Professor J. J. K. Best, Dr A. A. Donaldson and Dr G. R. Vauchan for the CT scans, and Blackwell Scientific Publications for permission to reproduce *Fig.* 11.7 from *Clinical Neuro-ophthalmology* (Ashworth and Isherwood 1981) as *Fig.* 14.1

REFERENCES

Albert M. L., Reches A. and Silverberg R. (1975) *J. Neurol. Neurosurg. Psychiatry* **38**, 546.
Alexander M. P. and LoVerme S. R. (1980) *Neurology (NY)* **30**, 1193.

Bell R. A. and Thompson H. S. (1978) *Arch. Ophthalmol.* **96**, 638.
Bever C. I., Aquino A. V., Penn A. S. et al. (1981) *Neurology (NY)* **30**, 387.
Bourgon P., Pilley S. F. J. and Thompson H. S. (1978) *Am. J. Ophthalmol.* **85**, 373.
Brazis P. W., Biller J. and Fine M. (1981) *Neurology (NY)* **31**, 920.
Chamberlain W. (1971) *Am. J. Ophthalmol.* **77**, 250.
Cohen D. N., Salanga V. D., Hully W. et al. (1976) *Neurology (NY)* **26**, 455.
Critchley M. (1964) *J. Neurol. Sci.* **1**, 274.
Damasio A. R., Damasio H. and Van Hoesen G. W. (1982) *Neurology (NY)* **32**, 331.
Devaney K. D. and Johnson H. A. (1980) *J. Gerontol.* **35**, 836.
Fisher C. M. (1980) *Arch. Neurol.* **37**, 502.
Geschwind N. (1965) *Brain* **88**, 585.
Goldhammer Y. (1982) Communication to International Society of Neuro-ophthalmology, Bermuda.
Green G. J. and Lessell S. (1977) *Arch. Ophthalmol.* **95**, 121.
Greenblatt S. H. (1973) *Brain* **96**, 307.
Harriman D. G. F. and Garland H. (1968) *Brain* **91**, 401.
Heilman K. M. and Valensteim E. (1979) *Ann. Neurol.* **5**, 166.
Ito Y., Miledi R., Vincent A. et al. (1978) *Brain* **101**, 345.
Kinsbourne M. and Warrington E. K. (1963) *Brain* **86**, 697.
L'Hermitte F. and Beauvois M. F. (1973) *Brain* **96**, 695.
Loewenfeld I. F. and Thompson H. S. (1981) *Ann. Neurol.* **10**, 275.
Malone D. R., Morris H. C., Kay M. C. et al. (1982) *J. Neurol. Neurosurg. Psychiatry* **45**, 820.
Meadows J. C. (1974a) *J. Neurol. Neurosurg. Psychiatry* **37**, 489.
Meadows J. C. (1974b) *Brain* **97**, 615.
Meyer B. C. (1947) *Arch. Neurol. Psychiat.* **57**, 464.
Osserman K. E. and Genkins G. (1966) *Ann. N. Y. Acad. Sci.* **135**, 312.
Ottomo M. and Heimburger R. F. (1980) *J. Neurosurg.* **53**, 97.
Pevzner S., Borristein B. and Loewenthal M. (1962) *J. Neurol. Neurosurg. Psychiatry* **25**, 336.
Raymond L. A. and Tew J. (1978) *J. Neurol. Neurosurg. Psychiatry* **41**, 83.
Russell R. W. R. and Pennybacker J. (1961) *J. Neurol. Neurosurg. Psychiatry* **24**, 1.
Ruttern F. (1947) *Monatschr. f. Psychiat. u. Neurol.* **114**, 265.
Scheie H. G. (1940) *Arch. Opthalmol.* **24**, 225.
Seybold M. E., Yoss R. E., Hollenhorst R. W. et al. (1971) *Neurology* **21**, 233.
Shipkin P. M., Gray B. S., Daroff R. B. et al. (1981) *Neuro-ophthalmology* **2**, 123.
Simpson J. A. (1960) *Scot. Med. J.* **5**, 419.
Smith S. E., Smith S. A., Brown P. M. et al. (1978) *Br. Med. J.* **2**, 924.
Thompson H. S. (1977) *Trans. Am. Ophthalmol. Soc.* **75**, 587.
Thompson H. S. (1978) *Arch. Ophthalmol.* **96**, 1615.
Vincent A. and Newsom-Davis J. (1980) *J. Neurol. Neurosurg. Psychiatry* **43**, 590.
Watson R. I. and Heilman K. M. (1979) *Neurology* **29**, 690.
Whiteley A. M. and Warrington E. K. (1977) *J. Neurol. Neurosurg. Psychiatry* **40**, 395.
Wilson S. A. K. (1906) *Brain* **24**, 524.
Wirtschafter J. D., Volk C. R. and Sawchuk R. J. (1978) *Ann. Neurol.* **4**, 1.

15. SOCIAL ASPECTS OF BLINDNESS IN OLD AGE
W. Wilson

GENERAL CONSIDERATIONS

As stated in Chapter 1, there is no internationally accepted definition of blindness. That commonly used is a corrected visual acuity not exceeding 3/60 or 10/200 Snellen in the better eye, or a limitation to less than 20 degrees of the visual field. However, many patients with a corrected vision of 6/60 or 20/200 are seriously handicapped visually, and it has been strongly urged that wherever possible the definition of blindness should be expanded to include those with this degree of visual loss, as is already the case in the USA.

That the definition should vary is understandable, since what can be considered a severe visual handicap varies throughout life. In the early years it is essential to have enough vision to profit from seeing and copying adults and other children, and to learn from moving about. By school age a much higher standard is needed to see writing on a blackboard and to read large print books, and soon the print of school books becomes smaller, and an even higher visual acuity is required. In adult life the visual standard is related to employment in a variety of jobs, each with its own visual requirement. In the elderly, vision is principally needed to maintain a home and, so as far as other disabilities permit, to preserve independence and to attend to one's personal needs (including moving about the house and in the street).

Contrary to popular belief, blind persons, while denied good visual acuity or a full visual field, are rarely unable to distinguish light and dark. The terms 'visually handicapped' and 'severely visually handicapped' might be more appropriate, but the term 'blindness', with its strong emotional appeal, is invaluable when raising funds for voluntary agencies, and is unlikely to be abandoned.

It is only after injury or a severe vascular incident that sight is suddenly lost, and most patients therefore have a period of adjustment. In the elderly the problem is usually that of slowly diminishing sight at a time of life when adjustment is especially difficult, and the need for it frequently resented. The psychological impact of becoming blind may often be profound, and can lead to a total loss of confidence. This is not helped if

156

relatives become overprotective, and others treat the elderly blind as though they were deaf or mentally abnormal. For the old in particular the management of daily chores such as shopping, housework, and the reading and writing of letters and documents all present problems. The latter may lead to the complaint of loss of privacy especially in financial affairs.

Since in developed countries 75 per cent of the blind are of retirement age (*see* Chapter 1), blindness makes its greatest impact on the elderly. Unfortunately the senses of touch and hearing may also be defective, and in addition many elderly blind may be confused. A geriatrician can be of considerable help to the ophthalmologist faced with the blind and disorientated patient. Will removal of a cataract promote return to a near normal mental state? Can the patient be expected to become independent after operation? The answers to these questions determine the advisability of surgery.

In the early days of the handicap both the ophthalmologist and the family doctor are in a unique position to help, the former because he knows the disease and the latter because of his special knowledge of the family and the home. However, the former may back away from aiding the blind, and the latter may be under too much pressure to provide practical assistance. Neither may be able or willing to undertake the time-consuming task. For the elderly the geriatrician may be the best placed to co-ordinate the resources needed to undertake the rehabilitation of the recently blind and maximize their independence.

LOW VISION AIDS

An elderly patient may not complain of poor vision, but may accept it as an inevitable part of growing old. As long as he can discern visual clues, these may be used with great resourcefulness and tenacity. Many patients of high intelligence and strong will, who were avid readers or pursued absorbing hobbies, will insist on attempting to continue with these. With depressing regularity the elderly patient clings to the fallacy that the 'eyes' should be preserved by not being used. They must be counselled not to sit in the dark avoiding all visual stimuli, but should rather be encouraged to make every use of the visual aids described.

In the first instance the patient with poor vision should be examined to determine whether glasses will help in any way. The time-honoured limit of +3 dioptres for near addition for reading cannot be applied to a patient who has to bring letters and numbers closer than 33 cm for them to be interpreted. If print must be brought to 10 cm for reading, the addition must be +10 dioptres, if to 4 cm +25 dioptres. Since for technical reasons print cannot be brought closer than 8 cm for binocular vision, the upper limit for a binocular addition is +12 dioptres.

Telescopic lenses are the only optical means of bringing objects close to an eye which cannot resolve detailed images at a distance. Galilean telescopes use a lens system combining a high minus lens with a weaker plus lens. The combination enlarges the retinal image of distant, intermediate and near objects. If telescopic systems are used as near aids, they must have reading additions for the required working distance attached to them or built into the front of the lens system.

Interests and hobbies such as cooking, selecting clothes, typing, writing and watching television are often more important than reading. In general central scotomas respond well to magnification provided that the peripheral retina is normal. Myopes can continue to read without a correction long after deterioration in distance vision. For instance, a patient with -12 dioptres of myopia can achieve 3x magnification at the natural near point, and one with -20 dioptres 5x.

A spectacle-mounted aid has the widest field of the low vision aids especially in the lower powers, but the close and fixed reading distance is a marked disadvantage. If the patient rejects a spectacle-mounted aid, a hand-held model may be recommended. One hand must support the reading material while the other supports the lens. Each hand is thus used for a separate adjustment, of the distance of the print from the eye and of the distance of the lens from the page. Both can be varied at will, an impossibility with a spectacle-mounted lens. A hand magnifier is useful for spotting objects such as telephone numbers, price tags and menu cards. Elderly patients with tremor or arthritis may prefer a stand magnifier; although the field is smaller, the stand can be moved along the page.

In considering reading material it must be remembered that patients with reduced vision always prefer good contrast to high magnification. For good contrast jet black print is needed on clean white paper with the letters well spaced. Lighting must be good, and free from glare; a multiposition lamp with an opaque shade is to be preferred. Magnification reduces contrast, and creates a conflict between the printed work and the background paper. Thus daily papers, normally printed on poor quality 'grey' paper, are a great source of visual difficulty, particularly to the visually handicapped elderly.

Relatives and friends of the visually handicapped should be encouraged to use fibre-tipped pens and black ink, and should write or print large letters and numbers. Finally, closed-circuit television giving a magnification of 50x enables some of the blind to read, but the equipment is expensive and is only of benefit to the highly motivated.

It is important to realize that legible handwriting may be preserved after many years of blindness, the principal difficulty being to keep the lines straight; the Royal National Institute for the Blind supplies special guides to enable the blind to sign documents and forms at the appropriate place.

SERVICES FOR THE BLIND

The talking book is perhaps the most important item of the welfare services for the blind. It is also available to visually handicapped persons not on the Register but certified by an ophthalmologist as having poor reading vision (N12 or less). With 55 000 subscribers, well over half the registered blind are members of the British Talking Book Service, which has close on 4,000 titles. The service is subsidized by the Royal National Institute for the Blind; many local authorities and voluntary agencies are prepared to help with the membership fee. Tapes, which can only be played on the special machines supplied to members, are sent to and fro by Freepost, and the machines are maintained by volunteers.

Talking magazines and newspapers are frequently organized by groups of volunteers. The former consist of items from local and national newspapers recorded on tape and supplemented by items of interest to the blind; they are often recorded on standard cassettes for use on commercial tape recorders. The tape is also a convenient method of exchanging news within a family.

Radio is a much better medium than television sound for the blind. The British Wireless Fund for the Blind was created to ensure that any blind person could have a radio together with a free supply of batteries. Both the BBC and the local radio present a weekly programme for the visually handicapped containing items of interest to the blind.

The telephone is another invaluable aid enabling the blind person to keep in touch with friends and relatives without leaving the house, to order food and services, and to summon help. A Telephone for the Blind service has been set up in some areas to help with telephone installation costs, but the running costs are usually expected to be met by the blind person.

BLIND REGISTRATION

Patients fear blindness more than any handicap and often attach themselves to an ophthalmologist for reassurance. They should be introduced to the social services for the blind, and in the UK can present themselves for blind registration at any time. However some resist any suggestion of registration, being reluctant to have their affairs looked into, or to appear to be accepting charity.

The general pattern of services for the blind is similar in many countries, but the method of gaining access to the benefits varies. Almost everywhere eligibility for help is achieved by inclusion in a register of blind or partially sighted persons, but responsibility for compilation and maintenance of such registers is not constant (*see* Chapter 1). They are the responsibility of the Social Services Department in England and

Wales, and of the Social Work Department in Scotland. These departments have a statutory duty to offer a wide range of services to blind people either themselves or through voluntary societies acting as their agents.

To be registered as blind or partially sighted is voluntary and need not be permanent. When duly completed by the ophthalmologist form BD8 in England and Wales (or form BP1 in Scotland) is sent to the Director of Social Services of the local authority concerned, and a qualified social worker then visits the patient to explain the range of local and national services available, and to establish the financial status and basic requirements of the registrant.

A Technical Officer for the Blind is assigned to each case to deal with the many problems created by blindness. He will visit regularly to advise on methods of cooking, cleaning, etc., and in overcoming the numerous hazards surrounding free and safe movement around the house. The blind person will be advised on the wide range of equipment available, such as clocks, barometers, thermometers etc. that can be read by touch. He is also able to provide instruction on the use of Braille and Moon type. Since in the elderly the sense of touch is poor, learning Braille is difficult, but some can be helped by the larger and simpler Moon type. Unfortunately there is no effective way of writing Moon type, and indeed instruction is only helpful to a small proportion of the elderly blind.

To venture outside the house may require the services of a Mobility Officer, who may be assigned to help with instruction and practice in the use of the long and the short cane. The former can give free and safe movement, and the latter can alert passers-by to lend a hand as needed. The stick is traditionally marked with a red band if the user is also deaf.

FINANCIAL BENEFITS

Most persons who become blind are forced to face increased financial burdens. In the UK blind persons whose income is so low that they qualify for Supplementary Benefit are entitled to a higher rate than those not registered. All blind persons (and the sighted spouse of a blind taxpayer if a joint return is submitted) are entitled to a special income tax allowance. This concession does not apply to those receiving non-taxable Government pensions for blindness resulting from war injury or a service-related cause. Both these benefits are only available to the blind and not to the partially sighted.

Despite the difficulties the blind have in travelling even a short distance, they are not entitled under existing regulations to a mobility allowance unless they also suffer from other physical or mental disabilities which render them unable to walk. Nor does blindness, unless complicated by very serious additional factors, entitle its victim to qualify for a Constant Attendance Allowance.

In most advanced countries travel concessions are available for a blind person or his guide on most local and some long distance buses and undergrounds. In the UK the blind person and his guide pay only one fare on the railways, but this only applies after he has purchased a railcard. On most international air routes the blind traveller and his companion must pay the full fare.

FUTURE DEVELOPMENTS

It must be conceded that the blind incur considerably increased expenditure by being dependent on others at a time when labour costs have never been higher. First priority must therefore be given to this aspect of the problem. Although Social Service programmes and private organizations have gone some way to reducing the additional costs imposed by blindness, only the payment of a realistic blindness allowance to all registered blind persons will suffice, as is already done in some countries.

There is also room for improvement in the attitudes of some ophthalmologists and geriatricians, who have only a sketchy idea of the social services for the blind and have tended to regard blindness as an endpoint, with strong overtones of failure. Voluntary help through organized charities and good neighbours—invaluable to those in need and often to those who serve—will always be required to augment the general services and to enable the elderly blind to be a respected and useful part of society.

USEFUL LITERATURE

The Royal National Institute for the Blind (224 Great Portland Street, London W1N 6AA) publishes a catalogue (and price list) of RNIB aids and games for the blind, and a short pamphlet entitled 'Information for People losing their Sight'.

Index